Management and
Treatment of
**BENIGN
CUTANEOUS
VASCULAR
LESIONS**

Oon Tian Tan, M.D.

Dermatology and Laser Surgery
Haddon Hall
Boston, Massachusetts

Management and Treatment of
BENIGN CUTANEOUS VASCULAR LESIONS

1992

LEA & FEBIGER
Philadelphia   London

Lea & Febiger
Box 3024
200 Chester Field Parkway
Malvern, Pennsylvania 19355
U.S.A.

Library of Congress Cataloging in Publication Data
Management and treatment of benign cutaneous
    vascular lesions / [edited by]Oon Tian Tan.
        p. cm.
    Includes index.
    ISBN 0-8121-1489-2
    1. Hemangiomas—Treatment. 2. Birthmarks
—Treatment. 3. Skin—Blood vessels—Laser
surgery. I. Tan, Oon T.
    [DNLM: 1. Hemangioma—therapy 2. Lasers
—therapeutic use. 3. Light Coagulation.
4. Skin Neoplasms—therapy. QZ 340 M266]
RL793.M36 1992
616.99'377—dc20   92-11546
                                              CIP

Reprints of chapters may be purchased from Lea &
Febiger in quantities of 100 or more. Contact Sally
Grande in the Sales Department.

Foreword

Few medical entities have attracted as much attention and created as much therapeutic confusion as the heterogeneous group known as benign cutaneous vascular lesions.

The conspicuous appearance of these lesions on the face, eyelids, lips, hands, and exposed areas has occasioned much speculation and superstition. In antiquity, individuals so afflicted were thought to have been touched by the hand of God or marked by the Devil, depending upon the persuasion of the observers. One of the most damaging concepts arising from these beliefs was that such afflictions were divine retribution for sins of the parents. More recent etiologic myths indict dietary discretions, drug use, and a host of other possible causative factors. One of the most current comments advanced by parents and patients is: "That mark is where the doctor put his forceps during delivery." In our litigious society the tremors generated by such remarks are palpable.

With the ready accessibility of such a dramatic and discomforting lesion, it is inevitable that treatments employed have been aggressive and varied. Early physicians described the application of hot metal as an actual cautery, incisions to "bleed out" the lesion, dermabrasion with salt and caustic agents, multiple sutures and ligatures, injections of corrosive agents, freezing by a wide variety of modalities (including exposure to the elements, ice, carbon dioxide snow, liquid nitrogen), injection of steroids, injection of anticoagulants, and irradiation. As usual, the multiplicity of remedies is compelling evidence of the lack of adequate efficacy and satisfaction with any.

The advent of the laser in the early 1960s provided yet another treatment possibility. Initial clinical work with the carbon dioxide laser was followed by studies with argon and neodymium:YAG wavelengths. Such early studies were important but empiric and were characterized by some as the "burn and learn" period of laser dermatologic applications.

Because of the intense emotional trauma to which children with vascular facial lesions were subjected, much early laser therapeutic effort was devoted to treatment in this age group. It was soon found that results of treatment, especially in flat, lighter-colored lesions, were variable, and the amount of scarring was unacceptable. As a result of these observations, many laser treatment protocols excluded patients under 12 years of age. This situation, unfortunately, prevented assistance to those individuals who most needed to ·avoid a future punctuated by untoward attention and discrimination.

Results of laser treatment of cutaneous vascular lesions in adults were much better, but their outcomes were still imperfect. Flat, lighter-colored lesions could sometimes be improved upon with the occasional complication of scarring or hypopigmentation. Elevated, dark nodular lesions responded much better to the application of the argon laser, with the outcome of flattening, lightening in color, and an acceptable rate of scarring. Some reviews of patients' perceptions of outcomes of their treatment indicated that most adult patients felt that their appearance had been improved, but that they were still concerned about color remaining at the site of the lesion and/or scarring and hypopigmentation. While CO_2, argon, and Nd:YAG lasers provided acceptable and useful treatment in many cases, it became obvious that additional refinements and improvements were necessary, especially to help young patients and those with flat, pink lesions.

The next important step in improving results involved careful investigation of mechanisms and results of laser-tissue interaction. For instance, it became evident from pathologic studies of specimens from patients treated with the argon laser that a fairly uniform and nonspecific type of thermal injury had occurred with results dependent upon the presence or absence of post-treatment infection or abnormalities of wound healing.

The search then turned to the characterization of laser absorption by specific elements of the skin, especially hemoglobin, melanin, and the microvasculature. Effects of wavelength, pulse frequency and duration, repetition rate, and spot size were identified along with important tissue factors such as chromophores, coefficients of absorption, thermal relaxation times, and a host of other determinants.

All this investigative activity focused upon the ultimate goal in the treatment of cutaneous vascular lesions—selective ablation or photothermolysis of all abnormal vascular structures with the preservation of normal skin architecture: "The color is gone and there is no scarring."

The editor of this volume, Oon Tian Tan, M.D., was one of the first to respond in this quest for a better understanding of the processes involved in laser photocoagulation and the development of techniques that would allow selective photoablation of targeted skin structures. This book, a collection of excellent contributions by authors well qualified in the investigation, management, and treatment of benign cutaneous vascular lesions, presents the overriding themes of (1) the understanding of mechanisms of laser and nonlaser effects on cutaneous vascular lesions and (2) the selectivity of obliteration based on the understanding and quantification of laser effects upon highly specific cutaneous targets.

Salt Lake City, Utah   JOHN DIXON, MD

Preface

The use of lasers has transformed the treatment of benign cutaneous vascular lesions. From the inception of these devices, the potential relevance was seen in many technologies, including medicine. The rapid technical development of lasers over the last two decades has produced in medicine an explosion of new applications as well as continual refinement and improvement.

Although the basic laser concepts and techniques are logical, interesting, and understandable, it is undeniable that in clinical applications they have been veiled with an aura of mystery. The field is so new that competing opinions abound, as technical and clinical issues overlap, causing difficulty in the objective assessment of different devices and methods. The resulting confusion and uncertainty, perhaps inevitable in a new field, is particularly seen in the parents of children with cutaneous vascular birthmarks like port-wine stain.

Physicians not actively involved in the research and development of this rapidly advancing field have also found it difficult to critically assess and appreciate the published data. They frequently have found themselves in the position of having to make treatment recommendations to their patients involving highly sophisticated techniques that not only are very specialized, but, in most instances, have developed since their training.

Thus, the purpose of this book is to provide: (1) a background to the technical and clinical entities involved in benign cutaneous vascular lesions; (2) some explanations and rationale for advocating and recommending specific approaches and techniques; (3) certain guidelines for patient management and monitoring; and (4) some insight into clinical and patient experiences during these treatment procedures.

Undoubtedly the research will continue, and experience teaches us that the "last word" is not in. Nevertheless, even now, the developments in the treatment of cutaneous vascular lesions have been among the notable success stories of lasers in medicine. Those working in the field feel privileged and stimulated by the ability to offer a treatment to the patients, to eliminate some of their negative feelings, and to enable them to have a brighter future.

The need to share not only the successes but also the limitations of the techniques and the lack of understanding of some of these disease processes has provided a well-rounded stimulus to the compilation of this book.

Boston, Massachusetts   OON TIAN TAN, MD

Acknowledgments

First, my personal thanks and gratitude are extended to all those who have contributed to this book. These individuals have spent endless hours ruminating over the problems associated with benign cutaneous vascular lesions, and together we have met and have had the opportunity to share a "healthy," diversified, interdisciplinary, controversial approach to solving some of the problems. Each author is an authority in his/her own right; hence, it has been a great privilege to have had the opportunity to compile their individual approaches and thoughts in this book.

Further, my acknowledgment goes to all those who have supported the research, those who have created an environment to enable this project to proceed, those who presented us with insurmountable challenges, and those who believed that we would be able to solve some of these problems. In particular, my family: To my husband, Tim, and our children, Kate and Nicky, who have not only shared in our success with pride but have provided strength and support through trying times. To my father, Beng San, whose continued questions have stimulated me to continue this work. Special thanks are extended to Horace Furumoto, Ph.D., who, in spite of technical difficulties, had the vision to appreciate the clinical problems, skillfully modifying the technology to solve them.

Last, to all the patients and their families who have constantly challenged us with their questions and their problems—without them and their constant support, none of this work would have taken place.

O.T.T.

Contributors

John A.S. Carruth, F.R.C.S
Consultant ENT Surgeon
Consultant Otolaryngologist
Royal South Hants Hospital
Southampton, England

Dean Crocker, M.D.
Professor of Anesthesiology
Boston University School of Medicine
Department of Anesthesiology
Boston City Hospital
Boston, Massachusetts

Douglas R. Fredrick, M.D.
Department of Ophthalmology
Children's Hospital
I Medical Clinic of Santa Clara Valley
San Jose, California

Martin J.C. van Gemert, Ph.D.
Laser Center
Academic Medical Center
Amsterdam, The Netherlands

Mitchel P. Goldman, M.D.
Associate Clinical Professor of
Dermatology/Medicine
University of California
San Diego, California

Amal K. Kurban, M.D.
Professor of Dermatology
Department of Dermatology
Boston University School of Medicine
Boston, Massachusetts

Pina C. Masciarelli
Senior Occupational Therapist
UMASS Adolescent Treatment Program
Westborough State Hospital
Westborough, Massachusetts

Joseph G. Morelli, M.D.
Assistant Professor
Department of Dermatology
University of Colorado Medical School
Denver, Colorado

John B. Mulliken, M.D.
Associate Professor of Surgery
Harvard Medical School
New England Birth Defects
Boston, Massachusetts

John W. Pickering, Ph.D.
Laser Center
Academic Medical Center
Amsterdam, The Netherlands

E. Steven Roach, M.D.
Director of Pediatric Neurology Services
Children's Medical Center of Dallas
Southwestern Medical Center
University of Texas

P.G. Shakespeare
Clinical Scientist
Director Laing Laboratory
Odstock Hospital
Saulsbury, England

Lois E.H. Smith, M.D.
Instructor of Ophthalmology
Harvard Medical School
Children's Hospital
Boston, Massachusetts

Timothy J. Stafford, M.D., Ph.D.
Associate Professor of Anesthesiology
Boston University School of Medicine
Department of Anesthesiology
Boston City Hospital
Boston, Massachusetts

Oon Tian Tan, M.D.
Associate Professor of Pathology
Boston University School of Medicine
Laser Research Laboratory
Boston City Hospital
Boston, Massachusetts

A.J. Welch, Ph.D.
Professor of Electrical and Computer
Engineering/Biomedical Engineering
University of Texas at Austin
Austin, Texas

William L. Weston, M.D.
Professor of Dermatology
University of Colorado Medical School
University Hospital
Denver, Colorado

Contents

Chapter 1   The Classification of Vascular Birthmarks

John B. Mulliken

Our understanding of cutaneous vascular anomalies has always been impeded by nomenclature. Bewildering nosologic systems have evolved, offering an array of admixed histologic and descriptive terms. Often the same word is applied to entirely disparate vascular lesions. The word "hemangioma" is the most egregious example, for it is misused, in a generic sense, to describe vascular anomalies of differing etiologies and natural histories. Confusion in terminology has been responsible, in no small way, for improper diagnosis, illogical treatment, and misdirected research efforts. Furthermore, interdisciplinary communication is limited in the field of vascular anomalies. Each medical specialty has its own nosologic jumble.

The classifications of vascular birthmarks used in the past, and like those for other diseases, reflect the methodologic obsessions of the time. These nosologic systems follow the historically familiar sequence of descriptive, anatomicopathologic, embryonic, and biologic. This chapter begins with a brief review of the history of classification of cutaneous vascular anomalies. Only by knowing where we have been can we know where we are and where we might be going.

Descriptive Classification

The earliest and most enduring terms for vascular birthmarks derived from the concept of "maternal impressions." From antiquity it has been commonly believed that if a pregnant woman's emotions were sufficiently affected during pregnancy, her fetus might feel the shock and so be imprinted with a skin blemish.[1] Thus, the resultant birthmark was said to resemble the object or circumstance that affected the mother's feelings. Another common explanation was that if the mother desired or refused certain fruits, her baby might be indelibly marked with lesions that looked like cherries, mulberries, raspberries, and so forth. Superstitious belief in maternal marking lingers to the present day. Such folklore is supported by nosologic terms based on brightly colored edibles, e.g., "strawberry hemangioma," "cherry angioma," "port-wine stain," and "salmon patch."

Mother was always blamed for the birthmark. Her indictment was buttressed further by Latin terms for vascular anomalies, such as *macula materna, naevus maternus,* or *stigma metrocelis.*[2] By the early nineteenth century, however, observant physicians became aware of clinical differences between the commonplace "mother's marks" and the rare, more dangerous, pulsatile vascular birthmarks. John Bell, Edinburgh surgeon, anatomist, and artist, first used the term "aneurysm by anastomosis" to describe arterio-venous malformation (AVM). In his monumental *Principles of Surgery,* he clearly described the progressive course of AVM and realized this was a separate entity from the banal *naevus maternus* of infancy.[3] In 1818, James Wardrop, another Edinburgh-trained surgeon working in London, correctly emphasized that *naevi materni* could be either cutaneous or subcutaneous in location, and keenly observed that either "could diminish in size."[4] Thus *naevi materni* were not to be feared so much as the more alarming vascular anomalies known as "erectile tumor" or pulsatile "fungus haematode."[5]

Classification of disease based on descriptive terminology is predisposed to inaccuracy and confusion, particularly in the field of vascular birthmarks. These blood-filled lesions all look very similar in various shades of blue, red, and purple. The next epoch of classifying vascular birthmarks was heralded by the microscope and the ascendancy of pathologic anatomy.

Anatomicopathologic Classification

Rudolf Virchow, the father of cellular pathology, did not miss the opportunity to focus his microscope on vascular anomalies. He called them all "angiomas" and categorized them, based on channel architecture, as "angioma simplex," "angioma cavernosum," and "angioma racemosum."[6] Virchow presumed that Bell's "aneurysm by anastomosis" was a combination of cavernous and racemose angioma. Furthermore, Virchow conceived that one type of vascular anomaly could transform into another by cellular proliferation or vessel dilatation. In short, he believed that "angiomas" were truly tumors in a cellular sense that grow by extension of new blood vessels. Wegner, Virchow's onetime student, proposed a histomorphic division of lymphatic anomalies, remarkably similar to that of his professor: lymphangioma simplex, cavernosum, and cystoides.[7] Virchow's classifications would be perpetuated in textbooks well into the twentieth century. Virchow's angioma simplex became synonymous with "capillary hemangioma" or "strawberry mark." Later these terms were misapplied to "port-wine" stain with its capillary-sized channels. The histologic designation "cavernous" came, in time, to be indiscriminately assigned to vascular lesions that involute as well as to those that do not.

For the Armed Forces Institute of Pathology fascicles, Stout and Lattes gathered all vascular lesions, both acquired and congenital, under a compound heading of "hemangiomatoses and lymphangiomatoses."[8] Enzinger and Weiss, in their monumental text, list vascular lesions of disparate clinical behavior and etiology together as tumors, either "benign," "intermediate malignancy" (hemangioendothelioma), or "malignant."[9]

Any strictly histopathologic classification, without clinical correlation, has not proved to be useful in the diagnosis and management of patients with vascular birthmarks.[1]

Embryonic Classification

Beginning at the turn of this century, cardiovascular embryology seemed to flourish.[10-12] As a result of these investigations, vascular anomalies were envisioned as problems of faulty development, arrests at various stages of channel development.[13-16] Furthermore, it was hypothesized that the common hemangioma of infancy was an ''embryonic rest'' of angioblastic cells.[15]

These attempts at embryonic classification are conceptually appealing and superficially logical. When put to trial of clinical usefulness, however, embryonic systems failed to guide the management of a wide variety of vascular birthmarks.

Biologic Classification

A biologic classification, proposed in 1982, defined the cellular features of vascular anomalies of childhood and correlated these with physical examination and natural history.[17] We showed that, on the basis of cell kinetics and clinical behavior, there are two major types of vascular anomalies in infancy: hemangiomas, lesions demonstrating endothelial hyperplasia; and malformations, lesions with normal endothelial turnover (Table 1-1).[17]

There is no useful classification without properly defined terms. The Greek noun suffix ''-oma'' denotes a swelling or tumor. In modern usage, a tumor is characterized by cellular hyperplasia. This semantic refinement is crucial to a precise nosology for vascular anomalies.

The unmodified noun ''hemangioma'' should be restricted to a lesion of vascular origin that grows by cellular proliferation. This term is synonymous with older terms for this most common tumor of infancy: ''capillary,'' ''strawberry,'' or ''juvenile'' hemangioma, or ''benign hemangioendothe-

Table 1-1. Biologic Classification of Vascular Birthmarks

Hemangioma	Malformation
Proliferative phase	Capillary: CM
Involutive phase	Lymphatic: LM
	Venous: VM
	Arterial: AM
	Combined: CLM
	CVM
	LVM
	AVM

lioma.'' Hemangioma is, indeed, a neoplasm, the result of proliferation of endothelium (and other cell types) within any organ system, most commonly the skin. The proliferation of hemangiomas to establish a large cellular mass necessitates pari pasu the formation of new feeding and draining vascular channels (the proliferative phase). These vessels, within and around the hemangioma, do not constitute an associated vascular malformation. However, flow within a large hemangioma, and particularly an hepatic hemangioma, can give the clinical and angiographic appearance of arteriovenous shunting, thus mimicking a fast-flow type of vascular malformation. Hemangioma has a remarkable biologic characteristic that distinguishes it from most neoplasms, viz., spontaneous regression (the involutive phase).

Malformations make up the second major category of cutaneous vascular lesions (Table 1–1). These are vascular channel abnormalities, errors of morphogenesis. The dysmorphic channels exhibit a normal rate of endothelial turnover throughout their natural history. Vascular malformations are, by definition, congenital, and many thus are visible at birth. Certain types of vascular malformation, however, go undetected at birth, only to manifest themselves during adolescence or adulthood. Thus, the designation ''acquired'' for a vascular lesion must be used with caution. Malan struggled with the terminology, considering whether these anomalies were more properly termed ''angiodysplasias.''[15] The term ''malformation'' denotes an intrinsic abnormality in the development within an organ. The word ''dysplasia'' denotes abnormal development of a particular tissue (dyshistogenesis) at a later stage of embryogenesis and its anatomic result.[18] Unfortunately, lack of understanding of etiology and pathogenesis makes it difficult to distinguish ''malformation'' from ''dysplasia'' in any discussion of vascular anomalies. The presumption is that the vascular anlage is intrinsically abnormal; therefore the term ''malformation'' is preferred.

Vascular malformations are anatomically subdivided into the following groups, based on the predominant channel anomaly: capillary malformation (CM), lymphatic malformation (LM), venous malformation (VM), and arterial malformation (AM). Combined channel malformations occur commonly, e.g., capillary-lymphatic (CLM), capillary-venous (CVM), lymphaticovenous (LVM), and arteriovenous (AVM).

Characteristics That Distinguish Hemangioma From Vascular Malformation

The vast majority of vascular birthmarks can be properly categorized by history and physical examination.[19,20] For some infants, the physician must honestly admit to the parents that another examination, a few months later, may be necessary before the vascular abnormality can be accurately diagnosed. Deep-seated cutaneous lesions may be ambiguous; in these instances radiologic evaluation may be indicated. One must always be wary whenever an infant presents with a rapidly growing soft-tissue mass, particularly a lesion that feels unusually firm. Sarcoma lurks in the list of differential diagnoses.

Fig. 1–1. *A*. Newborn infant with faint macular patch left forehead. ***B*.** At 6 months of age, the forehead hemangioma is growing disproportionately to the child.

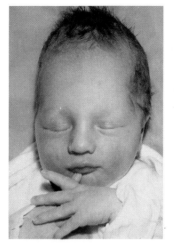

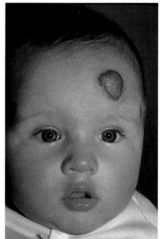

A   B

Clinical Differences

Hemangioma. A hemangioma is usually not seen in the newborn nursery; most manifest during the first to fourth week of life (Figs. 1–1, 1–2). The initial sign of a nascent hemangioma is either an erythematous macular patch, a blanched spot, or a localized telangiectasia, surrounded by a pale halo.[21,22] Rarely is a fully grown hemangioma seen at birth. Deep, subcutaneous, or muscular hemangiomas may not manifest as a cutaneous mass until the second to third month of life. A hemangioma may grow as a single localized tumor or may proliferate simultaneously in multiple sites, anywhere in the body. Approximately 80% of hemangiomas present as a single lesion; 20% of affected infants have more than one hemangioma (Fig. 1–3).[23] Multiple cutaneous lesions raise a suspicion for visceral hemangiomas. Female infants are more likely to have a hemangioma than males; the gender ratio is 3:1.[19,24] The incidence is higher in caucasian infants (10 to 12% by one year) than in other racial groups.[25]

The hemangioma's hallmark is rapid neonatal growth. If cellular proliferation begins in the superficial dermis, the skin becomes raised, finely

Fig. 1–2. *A*. Two-day-old infant is apparently normal. ***B*.** At 3 months of age, an extensive hemangioma infiltrates the right face.

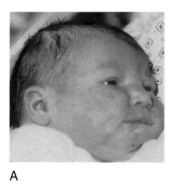

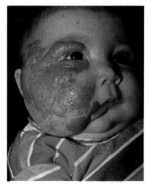

A

B

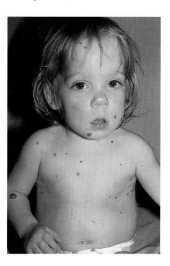

Fig. 1–3. Multiple, typically dome-shaped cutaneous hemangiomas. Visceral hemangiomatosis was not documented in this child.

bosselated, and with a vivid crimson color. If the hemangioma proliferates in the lower dermis and subcutaneous layer, without involving the papillary dermis, the skin becomes slightly raised, with a bluish hue. Often the overlying skin exhibits faint telangiectatic vessels (Fig. 1–4). Radial dilated veins also are commonly seen surrounding a hemangioma. Deep hemangiomas were once incorrectly labeled "cavernous"; or if the lesion involved both deep and superficial skin layers, the old term was "mixed" or "capillary-cavernous" hemangioma (Fig. 1–5). These microscopic adjectives "capillary" and "cavernous" are confusing and should be avoided. There is no such entity as a "cavernous hemangioma." The lesion is either a deep hemangioma or a mislabeled venous malformation. On palpation, a hemangioma feels like a fibrofatty tumor. The blood contained within a hemangioma cannot be evacuated by compression. These two physical findings usually serve to differentiate deep hemangioma from venous malformation.

Hemangiomas grow rapidly until 6 to 8 months of age. Thereafter, the parents often observe that the tumor's rate of growth has slowed, and now

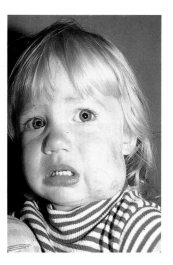

Fig. 1–4. Deep hemangioma of the cheek with telangiectasia in a 4-year-old girl.

Fig. 1–5. Hemangioma involving dermis and subcutaneous tissue of chest. Such a deep/superficial hemangioma should not be labeled "capillary-cavernous."

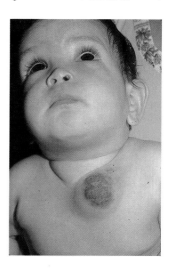

seems to be growing proportionately with the child. Soon, the early signs of involution can be seen. The once shiny crimson color begins to fade to a dull purple hue. In time, the surface assumes a mottled grayish mantle that seems to spread centrifugally toward the periphery of the lesion (Fig. 1–6). Now the hemangioma feels less tense to palpation. The parents may remark that their child is less fussy; or when the child cries, the hemangioma does not swell as much as it did previously.

Vascular Malformation. Cutaneous vascular malformations, by definition, are all present at birth. Not all of them, however, are obvious. A capillary malformation ("port-wine" stain) is usually apparent at birth, unless the child is erythematous, anemic, or darkly pigmented. Lymphatic anomalies are often noticeable at birth; most are present within the first year of life, and fewer than 20% are seen after one year.[26] Lymphatic malformations also can emerge in adulthood.[27] Venous anomalies may be present at birth, or they may manifest

Fig. 1–6. Extensive hemangioma of the left lower extremity and buttock in an 8-month-old infant. Note "graying" of surface, indicating the beginning of regression. Healed, previously ulcerated, area on the right buttock is a pale scar. Rare association with lipoma and tethered cord ruled out by ultrasonography.

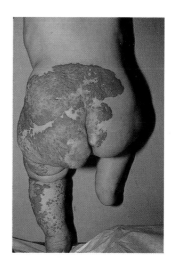

during childhood or adolescence. Arterial and arteriovenous malformations are usually not seen at birth. Like pure venous anomalies, they may appear late, often during puberty or pregnancy, or following trauma. There is no gender predilection in the vascular anomalies.

As a general rule, the vascular malformations grow proportionately with the child. As noted above, however, they may expand suddenly. For example, lymphatic anomalies often enlarge coincident with upper respiratory tract infections; they may present with cellulitis or with intralesional bleeding. Venous and arteriovenous anomalies often expand coincident with hormonal changes.

Each of the major categories of vascular malformation has a characteristic cutaneous appearance. A capillary malformation (''port-wine'' stain) is macular and sharply demarcated. The color ranges from pale pink to deep red, the hue deepening when the child cries, has a fever, or is in a warm environment. The pink flush, characteristic of infancy, gradually darkens to a deep red shade during middle age. The skin overlying a lymphatic malformation is usually normal. Occasionally, there is an associated capillary stain. The cutaneous (or mucosal) clue to lymphatic anomaly is tiny blebs or vesicles. A venous malformation is bluish, often tender to palpation, and easily compressible. Venous anomalies present in a wide spectrum, ranging from isolated skin varicosities, ectasias, or localized spongy masses, to complex lesions permeated throughout tissue planes. Arteriovenous malformations are not always so obvious; they may remain dormant for years. Early on, the overlying skin appears to be normal. In time, a pink macular blush appears in the skin overlying the fast-flow vascular anomaly. By now there is usually the telltale increased skin temperature. Later, the nearby veins become distended, particularly when the AVM is in an extremity. When an arteriovenous anomaly is ''active,'' palpation reveals a thrill, and a to-and-fro bruit is heard on Doppler examination. Arteriovenous shunting (steal phenomenon) diminishes nutritive flow to the skin, and ischemic episodes, even necrosis, may ensue.

Cellular Differences

Hemangioma. The rapidly growing hemangioma is composed of plump, rapidly dividing endothelial cells.[17] In addition, mast cells, known to play a role in neoangiogenesis, increase during the proliferative phase.[28] Mast cells subsequently fall to normal levels as the hemangioma's involution is concluded. As a hemangioma matures, it becomes organized into lobular compartments, separated by fibrous septa that contain large-caliber feeding and draining vessels. Autoradiographic studies of young hemangioma tissue demonstrate incorporation of tritiated thymidine into replicating endothelial DNA.[17] As the hemangioma regresses, the endothelial activity gradually diminishes. Tritiated thymidine uptake has been documented in a specimen from a 6-year-old child. Towards the end of one year, proliferation and involution seem to occur concurrently. Microscopic sections of older hemangiomas, well into the involutive phase, may exhibit scattered proliferative foci. In histologic specimens of children 2 to 5 years of age, there are fewer endothelial cells. The individual endothelial cells are less plump and appear less active. With time, there is a progressive deposition of perivascular, inter/intralobular fibrous tissue. The fully involuted hemangioma exhibits a ''cavernous'' appearance that can be histologically confused with a venous malformation.

Electron micrography reveals that a proliferating hemangioma is composed of plump endothelium that demonstrates characteristics of intracellular activity: convoluted nuclear membrane, swollen mitochondria, membranes of rough endoplasmic reticulum, and clusters of free ribosomes.[29] Multilaminated basement membrane is a pathologic hallmark of the proliferative-phase hemangioma.[29,30,17] Multilamination is not specific for hemangioma; it is also seen in other angiogenic proliferative disorders. Ultrastructural studies of involutive-phase hemangiomas expose interactions between mast cells and local macrophages, fibroblasts, and multinucleated giant cells.[31] There is also evidence of vascular degradation, e.g., endothelial death, discontinuity, and debris. The end-stage involuted hemangioma is composed of thin-walled vessels that resemble normal capillaries. The basement membrane remains multilaminated, and islands of fat and dense collagen are deposited in the perivascular areas.[31]

Vascular Malformation. Unfortunately, light microscopy of vascular malformations has not been particularly rewarding. At a cellular level, the endothelium of the various channel types appears quiescent. ''Port-wine'' stain is characterized by ectatic capillary to venular-sized channels within both the papillary and reticular dermis. The vessels are thin-walled and lined by flat, mature endothelium. Cellular turnover is undetectable in these capillary malformations.[17] Quantitative analyses by Barsky and associates show that a port-wine stain consists of an increased number of abnormally dilated vessels.[32] Immunohistochemistry demonstrates decreased to absent perivascular nerve fibers to the ectatic vessels.[33,34]

Venous and lymphatic malformations share a common appearance of walls of variable thickness. Some are quite thin, and others exhibit thickened walls. Often this mural variability is exhibited within the same lower-power microscopic field. Pale, acidophilic fluid is seen in LMs, whereas blood and the presence of thrombi characterize venous anomalies. The most complete descriptions of the pathologic anatomy of vascular malformations are by H.J. Leu of Zurich.[35–37] Prof. Leu has documented that degeneration of the walls in venous malformations is not a static process. In the early stage, the smooth muscle layer undergoes a reactive hypertrophy. Subsequently, under the influence of altered hemodynamics, the smooth muscle is replaced by collagen, resulting in a thin, fibrotic, inelastic vessel.

The arterial vessels in AVM are frequently dysplastic and hardly recognizable as arteries. They consist of thick-walled vessels with hyperplastic smooth muscle fibers within the media. The internal elastic lamina is typically fragmented, or the wall may be devoid of elastic fibers.[38,39] The smooth muscle is highly disorganized and not arranged in the usual circular pattern. The veins within an AVM appear ''arterialized.'' This may be a primary dysmorphogenesis or secondary to increased intraluminal blood pressure. These anomalous veinlike channels show reactive muscular hyperplasia and later degenerative changes such as fibrosis and atrophy of smooth muscle. In all the vascular malformations, the endothelium is flat and single layered. There is an occasional reference purporting to demonstrate endothelial hyperplasia in arteriovenous anomalies.[15]

Tissue-culture studies also demonstrate behavioral differences between hemangiomas and vascular malformations. Capillary endothelium, derived from infant hemangiomas, forms capillary tubules in vitro whereas capillary endothelium from vascular malformations is difficult to culture.[40]

Hematologic Differences

In 1940, Kasabach and Merritt described a 2-month-old infant with a large, rapidly growing hemangioma of the left thigh, who exhibited thrombocytopenic purpura and a prolonged bleeding time.[41] The coagulopathy was corrected coincident with spontaneous regression of the hemangioma. The term "Kasabach-Merritt syndrome" should be reserved for the profound thrombocytopenia that may complicate either a large hemangioma or extensive hemangiomatosis. The skin overlying the hemangioma is typically ecchymotic and shiny (Fig. 1–7). The coagulopathy occurs early in the postnatal period of rapid growth; the median age for admission to hospital is 5 weeks.[42] Thrombocytopenia, secondary to platelet trapping within the hemangioma, is the primary event. In time, fibrinogen levels fall and PT/PTT become markedly prolonged. This hematologic picture, though similar to a consumptive coagulopathy, is probably a secondary phenomenon.

Unfortunately, the term "Kasabach-Merritt syndrome" is often applied to the coagulopathy seen with large or extensive venous malformations. This hematologic defect is a true intravascular coagulation defect, with only mild thrombocytopenia and slightly decreased platelet survival. This is either a localized or disseminated intravascular coagulopathy, presumably triggered by stasis within the anomalous venous channels.

Radiologic Differences

For some patients, radiologic investigation may be necessary to differentiate a deep hemangioma from a vascular malformation. Furthermore,

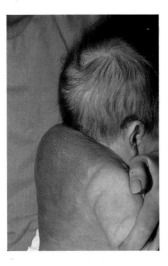

Fig. 1–7. One-week-old female infant with dark, ecchymotic, soft mass of back. Hematologic studies confirmed platelet consumption coagulopathy (Kasabach-Merritt syndrome), a rare complication of large and/or extensive hemangioma.

radiologic techniques may be needed to subcategorize a specific type of vascular malformation. Ultrasonography is the most cost-effective, and should be considered first. Ultrasonography (with Doppler flow study) differentiates slow-flow abnormalities, particularly LM from VM. But even an experienced ultrasonographer may have difficulty distinguishing an early proliferative hemangioma from an AVM; both are rheologically fast-flow lesions.[43]

Magnetic resonance is the most informative imaging modality for the study of vascular anomalies. Magnetic resonance imaging (MRI) demonstrates flow characteristics and portrays the extent of involvement within tissue planes. MRI can differentiate among fast-flow lesions, hemangioma, and AVM, as well as subcategorize the slow-flow lesions. Hemangioma demonstrates fast-flow in all spin-echo sequences (with presaturation), bright vessels on gradient-recalled echo scan with gradient moment nulling, and bright parenchyma on T1 and more so on T2 weighting. AVM is similar to hemangioma on MRI, but consists entirely of fast-flow vessels without intervening parenchymal stain. The various slow-flow anomalies can be differentiated on spin-echo sequences. Delineation of a lymphatic versus venous malformation or combined LVM is aided by gadolinium enhancement and repetition of the T1-weighted sequence.[44]

Computed tomography (CT) can detect contrast enhancement but cannot quantitate the rate of blood flow in a vascular anomaly. Dynamic scanning is needed to distinguish slow-flow from fast-flow lesions. CT does demonstrate the extent of tissue involvement and may best define the skeletal changes associated with vascular malformations.

Radionuclide scanning, e.g., with technetium-labeled red blood cells, will differentiate hemangioma from certain vascular malformations and from nonvascular soft-tissue lesions.[45] However, labeled red blood cell scintigraphy cannot subcategorize combined slow-flow anomalies or diagnose the relatively avascular lymphatic anomalies, and may confuse a proliferative-phase hemangioma with an AVM. Furthermore, radioisotope imaging fails to specify what tissues are involved.

Angiography is now rarely indicated except as part of treatment for an AVM by superselective embolization, or it may be performed prior to surgical extirpation of an AVM. Angiographic studies show a clear dichotomy between hemangioma and vascular malformation.[46]

Skeletal Differences

Growing hemangiomas rarely cause bone distortion or hypertrophy. Macrotia or maxillary/mandibular overgrowth may occur in the presence of large hemangioma. This phenomenon is presumably secondary to increased blood flow. Hemangioma may also cause a localized mass effect, e.g., depression of the calvaria, shift of the nasal skeleton, or enlargement of the orbital cavity.

In contrast, slow-flow vascular malformations are frequently associated with diffuse skeletal hypertrophy, hypotrophy, distortion, or elongation. The fast-flow arteriovenous malformations more often cause destructive interosseous changes.[47]

Subcategorization of Vascular Malformations

Vascular malformations are structural abnormalities, the result of errors in morphogenic processes that shape the embryonic vascular system between the fourth and tenth weeks of intrauterine life. These anomalies are almost always sporadic nonfamilial aberrations. There are instances of hereditary transmission of vascular abnormalities, particularly venous malformations. Familial capillary malformation of the central forehead[1] and rare pedigrees with Sturge-Weber syndrome[48] have been documented. Other vascular anomalies are well-recognized as hereditary, such as the Rendu-Osler-Weber syndrome, Fabry's disease, and ataxia-telangiectasia.

In the absence of knowledge of the etiologic factors and molecular mechanism underlying these vascular abnormalities, it is convenient to subdivide the malformations into the familiar anatomic groups, based on the predominant channel anomaly: capillary (CM), lymphatic (LM), venous (VM), and arterial (AM). The development of the embryonic vascular system is closely integrated, abnormalities in one part influencing the growth and morphogenesis of another. It is therefore not surprising to find vascular abnormalities involving more than one of the components. The combined channel malformations, commonly seen, are capillary-lymphatic (CLM), capillary-venous (CVM), lymphaticovenous (LVM), and arteriovenous (AVM) (Fig. 1–8). Furthermore, it is clinically useful to rheologically categorize vascular malformations as either slow-flow (capillary, lymphatic, venous, or combined forms) or fast-flow (arterial AM, arteriovenous fistulae AVF, or arteriovenous malformation AVM).

Capillary Malformation (CM)

These birthmarks have been incorrectly labeled "capillary hemangioma" or called by the Latin appellation "nevus (naevus) flammeus." The old tautologism "port-wine" stain deserves its hallowed position in our medical lexicon. The term capillary malformation (CM) has a familiar anatomic ring.

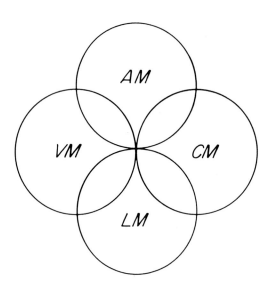

Fig. 1–8. Vascular malformations can occur as single-channel conformations. They can also present as combined anomalies, as simplistically represented in this diagram. AM = arterial malformation, CM = capillary malformation, LM = lymphatic malformation, VM = venous malformation.

Table 1–2. Classification of Vascular Malformations

Capillary (CM)
  Port-wine strain
    Sturge-Weber syndrome
  Capillary-lymphatic malformation (CLM)
    Circumscribed
    "Angiokeratomas"
  Telangiectasias
    Essential telangiectasia
    Rendu-Osler-Weber syndrome
    Ataxia telangiectasia (Louis-Bar syndrome)
  Cutis marmorata telangiectasia congenita
Lymphatic (LM)
  Localized
  Diffuse
Venous (VM) (CVM) (LVM)
  Localized
  Diffuse
Arterial (AM) (AVF) (AVM)
  Bonnet-Dechaume-Blanc syndrome
  Cobb syndrome
Complex-combined
  Regional
    Klippel-Trenaunay syndrome (CLVM)
    Parkes Weber syndrome (CLVM with AVF)
  Diffuse
    Maffucci syndrome (LVM, enchondromas)
    Solomon syndrome (CM, VM, intracranial AVM, epidermal nevi, osseous
          defects, tumors)
    Riley-Smith syndrome (LVM, macrocephaly, pseudopapilledema)
    Bannayan syndrome (AVM, LVM, macrocephaly, lipomas)
    Proteus syndrome (CM, VM, macrodactyly, hemihypertrophy, lipomas,
          pigmented nevi, scoliosis)

Port-Wine Stain. Port-wine stain (CM) should not be confused with the commonplace macular stain of infancy, known variously as "naevus flammeus neonatorum," "angel's kiss," stork bite," or "salmon patch" (Fig. 1–9A). These stains are commonly located in the glabella, eyelids, and nuchal regions; there is a remarkable tendency for these lesions to vanish within the first year of life. These fading macular patches may be more of a physiologic phenomenon than true dermatopathologic lesions. Histologic examination fails to demonstrate ectasia in the infant skin specimens; moderate ectasia of the subpapillary vessels, however, is seen in older children with persistent nuchal staining ("erythema nuchae").[49]

The literature is replete with references to port-wine stains in association with syndromes with dysmorphic features. Most of these citations are not port-wine stains, but cases of mistaken identity. Most of these vascular lesions are the ordinary fading neonatal stains, described above.[50] Furthermore, the majority of permanent capillary stains are not associated with other abnormalities (Fig. 1–9B). Capillary malformations are well known as markers in syndromes of vascular dysmorphogenesis. Many have eponymous

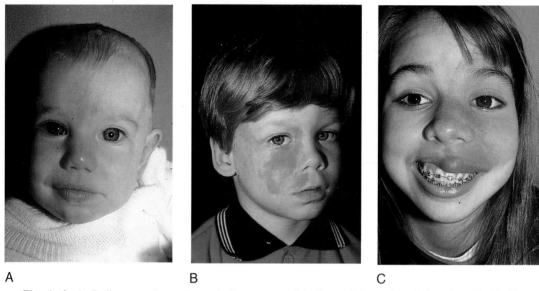

A   B   C

Fig. 1–9. *A.* Fading macular stain, typically seen on glabella, eyelids, and nuchal region. *B.* Capillary malformation (CM) in a patchy pattern within second trigeminal distribution. *C.* Sturge-Weber syndrome: capillary malformation with vascular anomalies of choroid and episclera. She has glaucoma OS; also note buphthalmos and hypertrophy of lip and maxilla.

labels. Sturge-Weber syndrome, as an example, consists of a capillary stain in the trigeminal (V1 or in combination with V2) dermatome, often with ipsilateral vascular anomalies of the choroid plexus and leptomeninges.[51] Cerebral angiography shows capillary, venous, and arteriovenous anomalies in this condition.[52] Children with these anomalies are at high risk for glaucoma. Soft-tissue and bone overgrowth, particularly in the midfacial region, is also commonly seen in this syndrome (Fig. 1–9C). Capillary malformation is also part of Klippel-Trenaunay and Parkes Weber syndromes, as discussed later. A capillary stain can be a "red flag," signaling an underlying developmental defect of the central neural axis. For example, facial port-wine stain may be seen with a unilateral arteriovenous malformation of the retina and intracranial optic pathway, a syndromic entity known as Bonnet-Dechaume-Blanc in the French literature[53] and Wyburn-Mason in the English literature.[54] In the cranium, a capillary stain may accompany an occipital encephalocele.[1] A capillary stain on the posterior thorax may be a clue to an underlying AVM of the spinal cord (Cobb syndrome).[55,56] A vascular blemish in the lower lumbar midline region frequently overlies occult spinal dysraphism, lipomeningocele, tethered cord, and diastematomyelia.[1]

Capillary-Lymphatic Malformation (CLM). Certain capillary stains have a rough, warty surface (hyperkeratosis). In the past, these lesions have been called by many names, e.g., "hypertrophic naevus flammeus," "verrucous hemangioma," and "angiokeratoma." Lesions that are present at birth and demonstrate vascular ectasia within both the dermis and subcutaneous tissue are more precisely called capillary-lymphatic malformation (CLM). These lesions have also been labeled "hemangiolymphangioma" and "lymphangioma circumscriptum" (Fig. 1–10).

Fig. 1–10. Capillary-lymphatic malformation (CLM) of the lower extremity in a little girl.

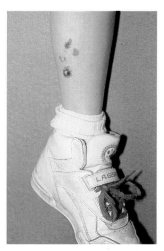

The angiokeratomas are clinically and histologically similar to CLMs. The vascular ectasia is limited to the papillary dermis.[57] In addition, the lesions usually appear in adolescence or later, i.e., they are "acquired" lesions. It is critical that there not be a precise differentiation between "acquired" and "congenital" vascular anomalies. It may take time before a structural abnormality of the vessels becomes manifest.

The angiokeratomas are best remembered by their eponyms and anatomic predilections: (1) Mibelli lesions on the hands and feet; (2) Fordyce lesions on the perineum; and (3) Fabry lesions on the trunk and thighs. It is difficult clinically or histologically to differentiate one type of angiokeratoma from another. Ultrastructural and three-dimensional reconstructions show a close resemblance between Fabry and Fordyce lesions. Both are believed to be developmental malformations of microvasculature and not the result of neoangiogenesis.[58] Angiokeratomas may have a genetic basis.[57] Biochemical abnormalities have been detected in Fabry's disease ("angioma corporis diffusum universale") and in fucosidosis.

Telangiectasias. The telangiectasias can be categorized alongside the capillary malformations, based on the caliber of the vessels involved. The major subcategories of malformative telangiectasias are: (1) ataxia telangiectasia (Louis-Bar syndrome); (2) essential (localized or generalized) telangiectasia ("angioma serpiginosum"); and (3) Rendu-Osler-Weber syndrome (hereditary hemorrhagic telangiectasia). The latter could also be designated as a fast-flow arterial malformation because AVFs and AVMs appear on mucosal surfaces and within many organ systems.

Cutis Marmorata Telangiectasia Congenita. Obvious in the newborn, the involved skin is traversed by a distinctive reticulated, serpiginous, depressed, deep purple colored vascular-like pattern. Sometimes there is ulceration of the involved skin (Fig. 1–11). Biopsy reveals dilated capillaries and veins in the dermis, and sometimes thin-walled, vein-like anomalies are seen in the subcutaneous layer.[59] Despite improvement, particularly during the first year, some degree of skin atrophy and vascular staining persists. Adult patients

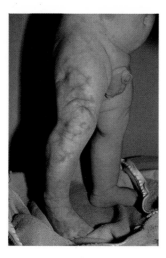

Fig. 1–11. Cutis marmorata telangiectasia congenita with distinctive depressed, reticulated vascular pattern.

exhibit with diffuse venous ectasia in the involved extremities. This peculiar pathologic entity could also be listed as a venous malformation.

Lymphatic Malformation (LM)

These malformations consist of localized-to-generalized anomalous lymphatic channels and cysts of various sizes and shapes (Fig. 1–12). In the past these anomalies have been referred to as "cystic hygroma"[60] and/or "lymphangioma."[61] The designation "lymphangioma circumscriptum" was introduced by Morris in 1889 to describe localized lymphatic anomaly with vesicular skin lesions. This latter intradermal lesion often presents in combination with capillary-sized channels (vide supra, CLM). Abnormal lymphatic channels are also seen in combination with venous anomalies, i.e., a lymphaticovenous malformation (LVM). The term "lymphangioma" is a misnomer because the suffix "-oma" implies a potential for growth by cellular mitosis and invasion. Some investigators believe that these anomalies

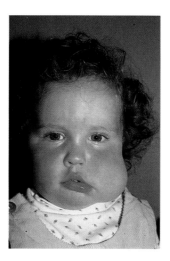

Fig. 1–12. Cystic type of lymphatic malformation (LM) of cheek.

Fig. 1–13. LM commonly associated with soft tissue and skeletal overgrowth. This is an example of macroglossia with typical hemorrhagic vesicles on dorsum of tongue.

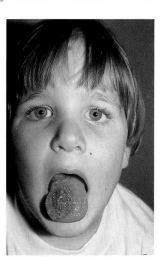

spontaneously grow by cellular hyperplasia.[62–64] However, tritiated thymidine studies of excised lesions fail to demonstrate endothelial hyperplasia.[17] It is more likely that lymphatic malformations expand secondary to fluid accumulation, cellulitis, or inadequate drainage of the anomalous channels.[65] There is no question that a lymphatic anomaly, once transgressed by surgical manipulation, has a remarkable tendency to regeneration, just as do transected normal lymphatics.

Lymphatic malformation is a common pathologic basis for a large lip (macrochelia), a large ear (macrotia), a large cheek (macromala) or a large tongue (macroglossia)[1] (Fig. 1–13). Skeletal hypertrophy and distortion accompany the majority of cervicofacial lymphatic lesions.[47] Limb overgrowth, both in length and girth, occurs in association with pure or combined lymphaticovenous anomalies of the extremities (vide infra, Klippel-Trenaunay syndrome).

Venous Malformation (VM)

Unfortunately, venous abnormalities are often included under the generic term ''hemangioma'' and erroneously labeled ''cavernous hemangioma,'' ''varicose hemangioma,'' or ''lymphangiohemangioma.'' These developmental anomalies of veins present in a wide spectrum, from isolated skin varicosities or ectasias, to localized spongy masses, to complex lesions involving multiple tissues and organs (Fig. 1–14A). Venous malformations are soft and compressible. Often small thrombi can be appreciated by the examining finger. Episodes of phlebothrombosis are common. Localized pain and tenderness on palpation are frequent complaints. Phleboliths, documented radiographically, are pathognomonic. The overlying skin/mucosa has a bluish hue. A combined cutaneous capillary-venous malformation (CVM) has a dark red-to-purple color. Combined lymphaticovenous malformation (LVM) exhibits superficial lymphatic vesicles and hyperkeratosis overlying the deep venous-channel anomalies. Stasis within a venous malformation may initiate localized or generalized consumptive coagulopathy.

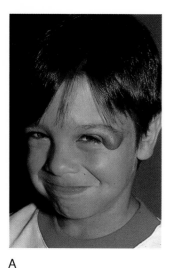
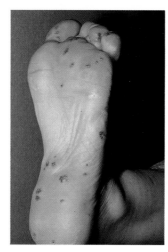

A   B

Fig. 1–14. *A.* Venous malformation (VM) involving glabella, eyelid, and temple. Venous anomaly distends with dependency, proximal compression, or Valsalva maneuver. *B.* Blue rubber bleb nevus syndrome.[69] Diffuse cutaneous venous anomalies that may be familial. This patient also has episodic gastrointestinal bleeding from bowel VMs.

There are syndromic designations for the rare, generalized venous malformations: diffuse phlebectasia of Bockenheimer;[66] Esau-Bensaude;[67] familial glomangiomatosis;[68] and blue rubber bleb nevus syndrome[69] (Fig. 1–14B).

Arterial Malformation (AM) (AVF) (AVM)

The fast-flow anomalies can be subdivided as follows:

(1) Arterial malformation (AM)—aneurysm, ectasia, or coarctation.

(2) Arteriovenous fistulas (AVF)—localized hemodynamically active shunts from large (truncal) arterial branches.

(3) Arteriovenous malformation (AVM)—a myriad of microscopic fistulas, diffuse or localized, the latter with a ''nidus'' of abnormal intercalated tissue.

Arterial malformations are rarely seen at birth; typically years pass before the ominous signs and symptoms of high flow become manifest. Some lesions lie hidden beneath an innocent-appearing cutaneous capillary stain (Fig. 1–15).

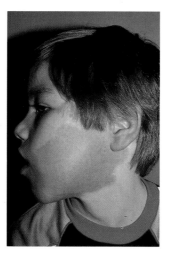

Fig. 1–15. Pink stain of left cheek overlies an arteriovenous malformation (AVM) of the mandible.

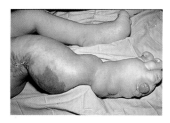

Fig. 1–16. Klippel-Trenaunay syndrome or capillary-lymphatico-venous malformation (CLVM) with soft tissue and skeletal overgrowth.

Complex Combined Malformations

The embryonic development of the vascular system is closely integrated with the morphogenesis of other mesenchymal tissues. Therefore, it is not surprising that vascular malformations occur with more than one type of channel component (arteries, capillaries, lymphatics, and veins). Associated overgrowth of soft tissue and bone elements is a common finding. The combination of slow-flow vascular malformations and gigantism is best known by eponymous syndromic designations. Sturge-Weber syndrome, for example, denotes vascular anomalies of the skin and central nervous system, possibly related to an error of morphogenesis of the cephalic neural crest.[51] Klippel-Trenaunay syndrome[70] should be categorized as a combined capillary-lymphatic-venous malformation (CLVM) in association with limb hypertrophy (and rarely hypotrophy) in length and/or girth (Fig. 1–16). In the majority of patients, the lower limb is involved, usually unilaterally. In some patients the upper limb alone is implicated. Bilateral or truncal involvement may also occur. The cutaneous birthmark of Klippel-Trenaunay syndrome is a macular capillary malformation (port-wine stain), or it may be studded with vascular nodules (cutaneous lymphatic/venous vesicles).

The Parkes Weber syndrome is a combined capillary-lymphatic-venous anomaly of typically the upper limb, plus arteriovenous shunting.[71] Maffucci syndrome denotes the coexistence of exophytic venous anomalies with bony exostoses and enchondromatoses[72] (Fig. 1–17). There are also complex vascular anomalies in the subcutaneous tissues, usually venous, but some-

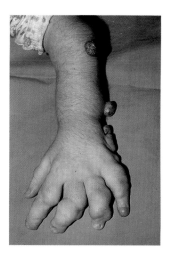

Fig. 1–17. Complex venous anomalies, enchondromas, and skeletal distortion, known as Maffucci syndrome.

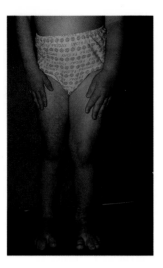

Fig. 1–18. Asymmetrical skeletal overgrowth (Proteus syndrome). Note axial hypertrophy of left upper/lower extremity and central toes with syndactyly and capillary stain of right leg.

times lymphatic in type.[73] In Maffucci syndrome, venous anomalies may also be present in bone, leptomeninges, and the gastrointestinal tract.[74]

There are many other described entities that lie within the spectrum of dysplasia of multiple tissues with vascular anomalies. The "epidermal nevus syndrome" includes patchy, linear, or sebaceous pigmented nevi in association with vascular anomalies of the skin and central nervous system and skeletal abnormalities.[75] The familial Riley-Smith syndrome combines macrocephaly with pseudopapilledema and multiple subcutaneous vascular malformations.[76] This is closely related to Bannayan syndrome, viz., macrocephaly with multiple subcutaneous lipomas, vascular malformations, and lymphedema.[77] The most inclusive designation is the Proteus syndrome. This is characterized by partial gigantism of the hands and/or feet, hemifacial hypertrophy, macrocephaly, with localized exostoses, pigmented nevi, thickening of the palms and soles, lipomatosis, and vascular malformations, both cutaneous and visceral.[78,79] Obviously, the dysplasia of cellular elements in all three germ layers has a wide and variable phenotypic expression. Asymmetric growth is, perhaps, the only constant feature of this syndrome (Fig. 1–18).

Conclusion

A classification of disease is ultimately useful only if it has diagnostic applicability, helps in planning therapy, and guides studies of pathogenesis. The schema of categorizing vascular birthmarks as hemangiomas or malformations is called "biologic" in the sense that it combines cellular features with clinical behavior. It is also a practical system, one that does not necessitate complicated diagnostic studies. An accurate medical history and physical examination (repeated, if necessary) permit accurate classification of cutaneous vascular anomalies in the vast majority of patients. If the diagnosis is in doubt, then ultrasonography and/or magnetic resonance imaging may be necessary. Radiographic imaging confirms the clinical subcategorization of vascular malformations as slow-flow or fast-flow anomalies, and is useful for determining the extent of anatomic involvement. Biopsy is indicated only if there is a question of malignancy.

References

1. Mulliken JB, Young AE. Vascular Birthmarks: Hemangiomas and Malformations. Philadelphia, WB Saunders, 1988.
2. Hooper R. Lexicon Medicum (Medical Dictionary), Vol 1. New York, Harper and Brothers, 1841.
3. Bell J. The Principles of Surgery. London, Longman, 1815, pp 456.
4. Wardrop J. Some observations on one species of naevus maternus with the case of an infant where the carotid artery was tied. Medico-Chirurgical Trans 9:199, 1818.
5. Dupuytren G. Leçons Orales de Clinique Chirurgicale Faites à l'Hôtel-Dieu de Paris, Vol 3. Paris, Baillière, 1839, p 225.
6. Virchow R. Angiome. *In* Die krankhaften Geschwülste, Vol 3. Berlin, Hirschwald, 1863, pp 306–425.
7. Wegner G. Ueber Lymphangiome. Arch Klin Chir 20:641, 1877.
8. Stout AP, Lattes RS. Tumors of the soft tissues. Washington, DC, Armed Forces Institute of Pathology, Fas 1, Second series, 1967.
9. Enzinger FM, Weiss SW. Soft Tissue Tumors, 2nd ed. Chapter 19, Benign tumors and tumor-like lesions of blood vessels. St. Louis, CV Mosby, 1988, pp 489.
10. Sabin FR. On the origin of the lymphatic system from the veins and the development of the lymph hearts and thoracic duct in the pig. Am J Anat 1:367, 1902.
11. Lewis FJ. The development of the lymphatic system in rabbits. Am J Anat 5:95, 1905.
12. Woollard HH. The development of the principal arterial stems in the forelimb of the pig. Contrib Embryol 14:139, 1922.
13. Reinhoff WF, Jr. Congenital arteriovenous fistula, an embryological study, with the report of a case. Bull Johns Hopkins Hosp 35:271, 1924.
14. DeTakats G. Vascular anomalies of the extremities. Surg Gynecol Obstet 55:227, 1932.
15. Malan E. Vascular Malformations (Angiodysplasias). Milan, Carlo Erba Foundation, 1974.
16. Szilagyi DE, Smith RF, Elliott JF, Hageman JH. Congenital arteriovenous anomalies of the limbs. Arch Surg 111:423, 1976.
17. Mulliken JB, Glowacki J. Hemangiomas and vascular malformations in infants and children: a classification based on endothelial characteristics. Plast Reconstr Surg 69:412, 1982.
18. Spranger J, Benirschke K, Hall JG, et al. Errors of morphogenesis: concepts and terms. J Pediatr 100:160, 1982.
19. Finn MC, Glowacki J, Mulliken JB. Congenital vascular lesions: clinical application of a new classification. J Pediatr Surg 18:894, 1983.
20. Mulliken JB. Cutaneous vascular lesions of children. *In* Serafin D and Georgiade NG (eds.), Pediatric Plastic Surgery. St. Louis, CV Mosby, 1984, pp 137.
21. Payne MM, Moyer F, Marcks KM, Trevaskis AE. The precursor to the hemangioma. Plast Reconstr Surg 38:64, 1966.
22. Hidano A, Nakajima S. Earliest features of the strawberry mark in the newborn. Brit J Dermatol 87:138, 1972.
23. Margileth AM, Museles M. Cutaneous hemangiomas in children: diagnosis and conservative management. JAMA 194:523, 1965.
24. Bowers RE, Graham EA, Tomlinson KM. The natural history of the strawberry nevus. Arch Dermatol 82:667, 1960.
25. Holmdahl K. Cutaneous hemangiomas in premature and mature infants. Acta Paediatr 44:370, 1955.
26. Gross RE. Cystic hygroma. *In* The Surgery of Infancy and Childhood. Philadelphia, WB Saunders, 1953, pp 960.
27. Nussbaum M, Buchwald RP. Adult cystic hygroma. Am J Otolaryngol 2:159, 1981.
28. Glowacki J, Mulliken JB. Mast cells in hemangiomas and vascular malformations. Pediatrics 70:48, 1982.
29. Höpfel-Kreiner I. Histogenesis of hemangiomas—an ultrastructural study on capillary and cavernous hemangiomas of the skin. Pathol Res Pract 170:70, 1980.
30. Iwamoto T, Jakobiec FA. Ultrastructural comparison of capillary and cavernous hemangiomas of the orbit. Arch Ophthalmol 97:1144, 1979.

31. Dethlefsen SM, Mulliken JB, Glowacki J. An ultrastructural study of mast cell interactions in hemangiomas. Ultrastruct Pathol 19:175, 1986.
32. Barsky SH, Rosen S, Ger DE, Noe J. The nature and evolution of port wine stains: a computer-assisted study. J Invest Dermatol 74:154, 1980.
33. Smoller BR, Rosen S. Port-wine stains: a disease of altered neural modulation of blood vessels? Arch Dermatol 122:177, 1986.
34. Rydh M, Malm M, Jernbeck J, Dalsgaard CJ. Ectatic blood vessels in port-wine stains lack innervation: possible role in pathogenesis. Plast Reconstr Surg 87:419, 1991.
35. Leu HJ. Einteilung und Pathomorphologies der Angiodysplasien. *In* Periphere Angiodysplasien, Schobinger RA (ed.). Bern, Hans Huber, 1977.
36. Leu HJ. Zur Morphologie der arteriovenosen Anastomosen bei kongenitalen Angiodysplasien. Morphol Med 2:99, 1982.
37. Leu HJ. Pathoanatomy of congenital vascular malformations. *In* Vascular Malformations, St. Belov, Loose DA and Weber J (eds.), Periodica Angiologica 16. Hamburg, Einhorn-Presse Verlag, 1989, p 37.
38. Leu HJ. Pathoanatomy of congenital vascular malformations. *In* Vascular Malformations, St. Belov, Loose DA and Weber J (eds.), Periodica Angiologica 16. Hamburg, Einhorn-Presse Verlag, 1989, p 37.
39. Mulliken JB, Dethlefsen SM. A preliminary morphologic study of an arteriovenous malformation and adjacent vasculature. *In* Vascular Malformations, St. Belov, Loose DA and Weber J (eds.), Periodica Angiologica 16. Hamburg, Einhorn-Presse Verlag, 1989, p 50.
40. Mulliken JB, Zetter BR, Folkman J. In vitro characteristics of endothelium from hemangiomas and vascular malformations. Surgery 92:348, 1982.
41. Kasabach HH, Merritt KK. Capillary hemangiomas with extensive purpura. Am J Dis Child 59:1063, 1940.
42. Shim WKT. Hemangiomas of infancy complicated by thrombocytopenia. Am J Surg 116:896, 1968.
43. Teele RL, Share JC. Ultrasonography of Infants and Children. Philadelphia, WB Saunders, 1991.
44. Meyer JS, Hoffer FA, Barnes PD, Mulliken JB. MRI correlation with biological classification of soft tissue vascular anomalies. Am J Roent 157:559, 1991.
45. Barton DJ, Miller JH, Allwright SJ, Sloan GM. Distinguishing soft tissue hemangiomas from vascular malformations using technetium labelled red blood cell scintigraphy. Plast Reconstr Surg 89:1992.
46. Burrows PE, Mulliken JB, Fellows KE, Strand RD. Childhood hemangiomas and vascular malformations: angiographic differentiation. Am J Roent 141:483, 1983.
47. Boyd JB, Mulliken JB, Kaban LB, Upton J, Murray JE. Skeletal changes associated with vascular malformations. Plast Reconstr Surg 74:789, 1984.
48. Tan OT. Personal communication, 1990.
49. Schnyder UW. Zur Klinik und Histologie der Angiome. Arch Dermatol 200:483, 1955.
50. Burns AJ, Kaplan LC, Mulliken JB. Is there an association between hemangioma and syndromes with dysmorphic features? Pediatrics 1991.
51. Enjolras O, Riché MC, Merland JJ. Facial port-wine stains and Sturge-Weber syndrome. Pediatrics 76:48, 1985.
52. Poser CM, Taveras JM. Cerebral angiography in encephalotrigeminal angiomatosis. Radiology 68:327, 1957.
53. Bonnet P, Dechaume J, Blanc E. L'anéurysme cirsoïde de la retiné (Anéurysme racemeux), ses relations avec l'anéurysme cirsoïde de la face et avec l'anéurysme cirsoïde du cerveau. J Med Lyon 18:165, 1937.
54. Wyburn-Mason R. Arteriovenous aneurysm of midbrain, retina, facial naevi and mental changes. Brain 66:163, 1943.
55. Cobb S. Haemangioma of the spinal cord associated with skin naevi of the same metamere. Ann Surg 62:641, 1915.
56. Jessen RT, Thompson S, Smith EG. Cobb syndrome. Arch Dermatol 113:1587, 1977.
57. Imperial R, Helwig EB. Angiokeratoma: a clinicopathological study. Arch Dermatol 95:166, 1967.
58. Braverman IM, Keh-Yen A. Ultrastructural and three-dimensional reconstruction of several macular and papular telangiectases. J Invest Dermatol 81:489, 1983.
59. Way BH, Herrmann J, Gilbert EF, et al. Cutis marmorata telangiectatica congenita. J Cutan Pathol 1:10, 1974.
60. Wernher A. Die angebornen Kysten-hygrome und die ihnen verwandten Geschwülste in anatomischer, diagnosticher und therapeutischer Beziehung. Giessen, G.F. Heyer, Vater, 1843.
61. Wegner G. Ueber Lymphangiome. Arch Klin Chir 20:641, 1877.
62. Goetsch E. Hygroma colli cysticum and hygroma axillae: pathologic and clinical study and report of twelve cases. Arch Surg 36:394, 1938.
63. Harkins GA, Sabiston DC. Lymphangioma in infancy and childhood. Surgery 47:811, 1960.

64. Bill AH, Sumner DS. A unified concept of lymphangioma and cystic hygroma. Surg Gynecol Obstet 120:79, 1965.

65. Willis RA. Pathology of Tumors, 3rd ed. London, Butterworth and Co, 1960, p 716.

66. Bockenheimer P. Ueber die genuine diffuse Phlebektasie der oberen Extremität. Festschrift FGE Von Rindfleisch, Leipzig 38:311, 1907.

67. Bensaude R, Bensaude A. D'angiome caverneux du rectum. Presse Med 93:1739, 1932.

68. Touraine A, Solente A, Renault P. Tumers glomiques multiples de tronc et des membres. Bull Soc Franc Dermatol and Syphil 43:736, 1936.

69. Bean WB. Vascular Spiders and Related Lesions of the Skin. Springfield, IL, Chas C Thomas, 1958, p 178.

70. Klippel M, Trenaunay P. Du noevus variqueux ostéohypertrophique. Arch Gen Med 3:641, 1900.

71. Weber FP. Angioma formation in connection with hypertrophy of limbs and hemi-hypertrophy. Brit J Dermatol 19:231, 1907.

72. Maffucci A. Di un caso di encondroma ed angioma multiplo contribuzione al a genesi embrionale dei tumor. Movimento Med Chir 3:399, 1881.

73. Loewinger RJ, Lichenstein JR, Dodson WE, Eisen AZ. Maffucci's syndrome: a mesenchymal dysplasia and multiple tumour syndrome. Brit J Dermatol 96:317, 1977.

74. Cremer H, Gulotta F, Wolf L. Maffucci-Kast syndrome. J Cancer Res Clin Oncol 101:231, 1981.

75. Solomon LM, Fretzin OF, Dewald RL. The epidermal nevus syndrome. Arch Dermatol 97:273, 1968.

76. Riley HD, Smith WR. Macrocephaly, pseudopapilledema and multiple hemangiomata. Pediatrics 26:293, 1960.

77. Bannayan GA. Lipomatosis, angiomatosis, and macrencephalia. A previously undescribed congenital syndrome. Arch Pathol 92:1, 1971.

78. Wiedemann HR, Burgio GR, Aldenhoff P, et al. The proteus syndrome: partial gigantism of the hand and/or feet, nevi, hemihypertrophy, subcutaneous tumors, macrocephaly, or other skull anomalies and possible accelerated growth and visceral affections. Eur J Pediatr 140:5, 1983.

79. Wiedemann HR, Burgio GR: Encephalocraniocutaneous lipomatosis and Proteus syndrome. Am J Med Genet 25:403, 1986.

Chapter 2   Modeling Laser Treatment of Port-Wine Stains

Martin J. C. van Gemert, John W. Pickering,
Ashley J. Welch

Laser treatment of port-wine stains (PWS) is a multidisciplinary endeavor. First, it involves art, that is, the skill of the clinician combined with the variability and unpredictability associated with each patient. A good clinician has an understanding of the physics and biology of the processes involved and varies the technique according to each individual patient. Naturally some unpredictability will exist among patients with respect to the chance of scarring, the final cosmetic outcome, and the required number of retreatment sessions. Second, laser treatment of PWS involves psychology, that is, the patient and clinician's subjective and objective assessment of the cosmetic result. A third factor is biology, or the body's response to the laser-damaged tissue. In the extremes, this may result in "ideal" wound healing or in scar tissue. Finally, there is physics, which is the subject of this chapter.

The physics may be divided into two parts. The first concerns the physical properties of the laser beam that is incident on the PWS, namely: wavelength, spatial distribution of power density, pulse duration (exposure or irradiation time), repetition rate, and spot diameter. Whereas production of laser light will not be discussed within this chapter, we will consider how this light interacts with tissue. This is the second part of physics, and it involves the dynamic sequence of events of light-tissue interaction, beginning with the spatial and temporal light distribution in the PWS skin tissue, causing a spatial and temporal rise in temperature and, finally, resulting in a spatial tissue damage distribution. The study of this process requires an anatomic model for the PWS and a mathematical model that can predict the optical, thermal, and biologic damage responses of the various PWS tissue components.

We shall consider four treatment parameters. The first is the wavelength or color of the laser light. Of particular interest are the wavelengths of the argon (488 to 515 nm), the frequency doubled Nd:YAG (KTP laser at 532 nm), the pulsed dye (normally 577 nm or 585 nm), the continuous wave dye (577 nm), and the copper vapor (578 nm) lasers. The second treatment parameter is the exposure time. This may be determined either by the length of the laser pulse—as is the case with the pulsed dye laser and lasers fitted with the Hexascan light delivery system[1]—or by the rate at which the light is scanned across the skin. The third is the irradiance (W/cm^2). This is the amount of light incident on the skin per unit area; it is the laser power divided by the area of the incident spot. Finally, we consider the influence of the laser spot diameter.

In order to make a prediction of clinical treatment outcome we must start with a statement about the clinical goal we want to achieve. In this chapter our goal is to irreversibly damage the wall of all ectatic PWS blood vessels and to maintain the integrity of all other skin constituents.

Next we must establish some criteria relating physical parameters like temperature rise to the skin's biologic response.

In this chapter we use the criterion that an ectatic vessel is irreversibly damaged, and will show subsequent ideal wound healing that leads to a normal skin vasculature, when the top of the vessel reaches a certain critical temperature (e.g., 70° C for 0.1 s exposure time[2]). Criteria of this sort are crucial to the modeling of laser treatment of PWS, but at the same time they are difficult to establish as there is currently insufficient knowledge of the relation between physics and biology.

This chapter is organized as four main sections. The first presents the assumptions and methods used for the analysis of laser port-wine stain interactions. These interactions are presented in the next section, which explains that the ideal laser parameters are: a wavelength of 577 nm or longer, but shorter than 590 nm; an exposure time longer than 0.1 ms and shorter than 10 ms; a laser beam diameter of 3 mm or more. The third section models the contribution of dermal blood to the color appearance of a PWS and confirms recent work by Tan et al.[3] that capillaries as deep as about 1 mm into the dermis need to be irreversibly damaged to remove the abnormal coloration. The next section is a final discussion with conclusions.

The authors have attempted to explain the assumptions, methods, and laser-tissue interactions as simply as possible, without mathematics, but with figures and tables to clarify as much as possible. For more mathematical details on modeling laser treatment of PWS, see the chapter of van Gemert et al. noted in References.[4] Some terminology used in this chapter pertaining to the physical distribution of light within the tissue is discussed in an appendix.

Modeling: Assumptions and Methods

PWS Anatomic Models

The first anatomic model of a PWS used in this chapter is shown in Figure 2–1A; it consists of a single ectatic vessel that runs parallel to the air-skin interface, of diameter between 0.03 and 0.30 mm, with a vessel wall thickness between 0.003 and 0.006 mm[5], and a hematocrit of 40%. The ectatic blood vessel is situated at a dermal depth (from the epidermis-dermis interface) between 0.1 and >1.0 mm. The skin consists of two layers, an epidermis with a thickness of 0.05 to 0.1 mm, and a dermis with a thickness of 1 to 1.5 mm. The subcutaneous layer (below the dermis) is not specified any further, as it seems unimportant for the analysis; that is, for laser PWS modeling the dermis has infinite thickness.

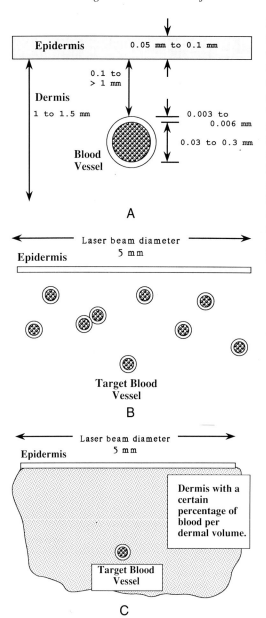

Fig. 2–1. Models used to simulate port wine stains: (a) Single-vessel model with a melanin filled epidermis of 0.05 to 0.1 mm, a bloodless dermis of 1 to 1.5 mm, a blood vessel of 0.03 to 0.3 mm diameter with endothelial cells of 0.003 to 0.006 mm thickness, and at a dermal depth of 0.1 to 1 mm. (b) Multiple-vessel model with numerous vessels of various sizes distributed throughout the dermis. One vessel is designated as the target vessel. A laser beam diameter of 5 mm. (c) Approximation to multiple-vessel model. For convenience the effect of multiple vessels is approximated by distributing the same quantity of blood contained within these vessels throughout the dermis (between 0 and 10% by volume of the dermis). For damage calculations a target blood vessel is placed within the dermis in the center of the laser beam.

We will show (as was first illustrated in 1981)[6,7] that a PWS model with only one single blood vessel (Fig. 2–1A) predicts 577 nm as the ideal wavelength for laser treatment.

The second anatomic model, which is more realistic than the previous one, consists of more than just one ectatic blood vessel such as shown in Figure 2–1B. It is obvious that not one single PWS model can be given in concurrence with clinical reality. It is essential that the laser beam diameter used for treatment be (much) larger than the average distance between vessels. In such a situation, a third anatomic model, shown in Figure 2–1C, is then appropriate and consists of one target blood vessel in a dermal environment that includes an average amount of blood (5% by volume, say).

We will show that models involving several vessels predict a wavelength of at least 577 nm but shorter than 590 nm as the best wavelength for laser treatment, depending upon dermal blood volume, laser spot diameter, and exposure time.

Clinical Goal and Ideal Laser Treatment

The clinical goal is to establish irreversible damage of the ectatic vessels without any damage to the other skin constituents. This goal leads to the definition of the ideal laser treatment of PWS, shown in Figure 2–2: laser illumination leads to coagulation and hence to occlusion of the ectatic vessel. Ideal wound healing is, several months later, for the ectatic vessel to be replaced by one or more "normal" capillaries.

How To Reach the Clinical Goal: The Unrealistic Case (If Nature Were Cooperative)

It is instructive to consider an unrealistic but ideal concept wherein only blood absorbs the laser light. Absorption of the laser light results in a temperature rise of the blood and consequent heating of the vessel wall by heat conduction. Obviously, the exposure time of the laser light must be sufficiently long to accomplish irreversible damage of the wall. Coagulation of red blood cells and vessel wall results in thrombosis and occlusion of the

Fig. 2–2. The biologic processes that we assumed for ideal wound healing. (a) Soon after laser irradiation. (b) The absorbed light within the vessel results in the coagulation of the vessel and irreversible damage to the endothelial cells. (c) Over the ensuing months the body replaces the damaged ectatic vessel by 2 or 3 normal-sized capillaries.

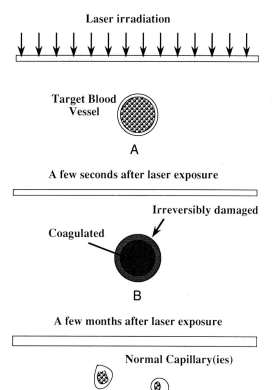

whole vessel without damage to the other skin constituents, provided that the laser exposure duration is shorter than the time it takes to conduct the heat a substantial distance into the surrounding dermis. Thus, the exposure time should be long enough to accomplish irreversible damage of the wall by heat conduction, and short enough to prevent conduction of heat too far into the surrounding dermis. Below, in the section on laser-PWS interactions, the ideal exposure time is shown to be longer than 0.1 ms and shorter than 10 ms.

How To Reach the Clinical Goal: The Realistic "Next-Best" Approach

Unfortunately, not only blood, but also all other skin constituents absorb laser light. Therefore, the "next-best," and realistic, approach to ensure selective vessel damage is to require the ectatic blood vessels to rise faster in temperature than any other cutaneous structure. This means finding laser wavelengths that are absorbed more by blood than by melanin and collagen, and that penetrate sufficiently deep into the skin to reach the deepest ectatic vessels requiring irreversible damage — that is, the deepest ectatic vessels that still contribute to the skin color (see section on modeling color appearance). The requirements for the laser exposure time are those of the previous paragraph, but with an upper limit that is determined by the time it takes the vessel to be just irreversibly damaged. Obviously, such an exposure time depends upon the laser power density used. Table 2–1 summarizes the assumptions upon which the "next-best" approach is based. To model these four treatment parameters requires a number of physical concepts, summarized in Table 2–2. Required, first, is knowledge of the absorption behavior of epidermal and dermal tissues as a function of wavelength. Second, a method is required to estimate how deeply into the skin light of a certain wavelength can penetrate, and what the resulting heat production, temperature, and damage distributions will be. The final result is a prediction of the depth of selective vascular damage in the skin, and whether that depth is sufficient for changing the stain color to that of normal skin.

Table 2–1. Assumptions Upon Which the "Next-Best" Approach Is Based

Wavelength	• Red blood vessels rise (much) faster in temperature than any of the other skin constituents during irradiation.
	• Penetration into the skin is sufficiently deep to reach all ectatic vessels that need treatment.
Pulse duration	• *Long enough* for sufficient heat to be generated within the red blood cells to irreversibly damage the ectatic vessel wall by heat conduction.
	• *Shorter* than the time taken for the hot blood vessel to damage a substantial dermal tissue volume by conduction of heat.
	• *Shorter* than the time taken for the other skin constitutents to be irreversibly damaged.
Irradiance	• Sufficient to achieve irreversible vessel wall damage under the constraints summarized in this Table.
Spot diameter	• *Large enough* for obtaining the maximum fluence rate per incident irradiance to reach the ectatic vessels deep within the dermis.

Table 2-2. Physical Concepts Required for the Treatment Approach

1. Absorption behavior of red blood cells (or whole blood), melanin, and collagen as a function of wavelength (see Fig. 2–8 and Table 2–3)
2. Spatial distribution of the fluence rate in the skin, i.e., depth of light penetration into the skin (see Figs. 2–3 and 2–9)
3. Contribution of a dermal ectatic capillary to the color appearance of the PWS
4. Propagation of heat by conduction inside the skin

Optical Behavior; Light Propagation, Fluence Rate, and Spot Diameter

The description of the propagation of light in an absorbing and scattering material such as tissue is mathematically complicated. It requires solving the transport equation of radiative transfer with the available absorption and scattering parameters of tissue. This has recently been done successfully by Monte Carlo numerical methods,[8,9] using measured absorption and scattering coefficients (in units of reciprocal length) and the anisotropy factor for scattering.

The resulting outcome is the spatial distribution of fluence rate (in units of laser power per area). The fluence rate is the locally available light intensity within the tissue, defined as the total amount of laser light power that crosses the surface area of an infinitesimally small sphere, located at the position inside the tissue that is considered, divided by the cross-sectional area of that sphere (see Appendix).

An important parameter that strongly influences the penetration depth of light in tissue is the laser-beam spot diameter. For *small* spot diameters—that is, for diameters smaller than, or approximately equal to, the average distance a photon travels between two scattering events (the scattering length, which is estimated as 0.2 mm for dermis at 577 nm)—occurrence of a scattering event implies that the photon is most likely to be scattered out of the (unscattered) beam. A subsequent scattering event will most likely *not* scatter that photon back into the (unscattered) beam volume again. The result is a virtually exponential attenuation behavior with tissue depth given by Beer's law, with the sum of absorption and scattering coefficients as attenuation parameters, and radial beam broadening with tissue depth. In contrast, for spot diameters that are much *larger* than the photon scattering length, scattering events inside the beam virtually do not result in depletion of photons, as only the most peripheral of photons can be scattered out of the beam. Therefore, photons "stay around" during scattering events, and one photon can, in principle, cross the surface area of that infinitesimally small sphere more than once. As a result, there is hardly any radial beam broadening with tissue depth, and the local fluence rate inside tissue can be larger than the incident irradiance. Figure 2–3 shows several fluence rate computations as a function of skin depth, for several beam diameters.

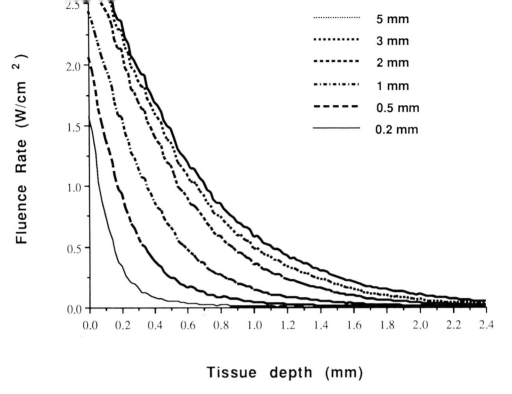

Fig. 2–3. The fluence rate within the skin below the beam center is influenced (owing to scattering) by the beam diameter. For the same incident irradiance (1 W/cm^2), the larger the beam (spot) diameter, the greater the fluence rate. These Monte Carlo calculations were made for a bloodless dermis at 577 nm using optical properties summarized in Table 2–3.

Thermal Behavior: Heat Production, Heat Conduction, and Tissue Damage

A local rise in temperature results from storage of heat in a local volume. It is a balance of, first, local absorption of photons that create a local volumetric heat production; second, conduction of heat out of that volume; and, third, conduction of heat into that volume.

Volumetric Heat Production. The local volumetric production of heat (in Watts per unit volume) is equal to the product of local absorption coefficient and local fluence rate. As an example, Figure 2–4 shows the volumetric heat production in the skin (Fig. 2–4C) along the center of the laser beam (Fig. 2–4A), with a fluence rate distribution obtained by Monte Carlo computations (Fig. 2–4B), assuming that, at 577 nm, the fluence rate distribution through the blood vessels is according to Beer's law with the blood absorption

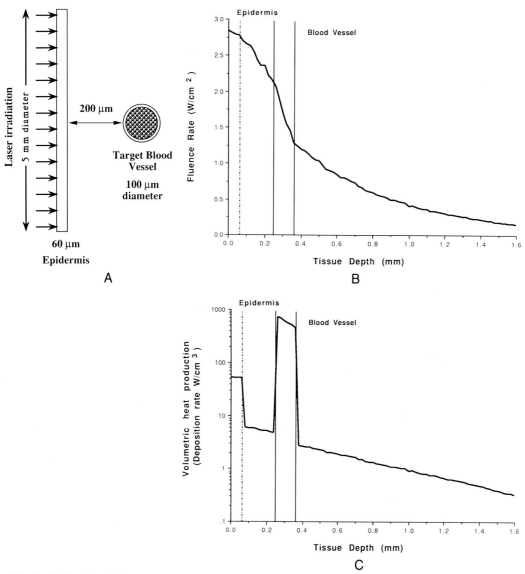

Fig. 2–4. The physical processes that occur during laser irradiation. (a) In the single-vessel model. (b) The incident light is absorbed by the tissue, particularly within the blood vessel and epidermis. (c) This absorbed light results in heat production: the (local) volumetric rate of heat production is equal to the product of (local) absorption coefficient and (local) fluence rate, and it is greatest in the blood vessel, less in the epidermis, and negligible in the dermis (note the logarithmic scale). Once more, these calculations are for 577 nm in a bloodless dermis, through the center of the laser beam, using the optical properties of Table 2–3.

coefficient as the exponential factor. (The optical properties used are given in Table 2–3, vide infra.)

Heat Conduction. Heat conduction, or the flow of heat from one location to another, requires a temperature gradient to exist between the two locations. If one location is at a higher temperature than the other, it will lose heat towards

Table 2–3. Optical Properties Used for Blood, Epidermis, and Dermis
(For blood absorption, see also Fig. 2–8.)

Wavelength (nm)	Absorption coefficient (mm^{-1})	Scattering coefficient (mm^{-1})	Anisotropy factor
Blood			
415	300.0	48.0	0.995
500	11.5	47.5	0.995
532	26.6	47.3	0.995
545	33.0	47.2	0.995
560	20.0	47.0	0.995
577	35.4	46.8	0.995
585	19.1	46.7	0.995
590	6.9	46.6	0.995
633	5.0	46.4	0.995
Epidermis			
415	3.30	80	0.743
500	2.40	59	0.760
545	2.00	50	0.780
560	1.90	49	0.785
577	1.85	48	0.787
585	1.80	47	0.790
633	1.70	50	0.820
Dermis			
415	0.35	32.0	0.743
500	0.26	25.5	0.760
545	0.23	23.0	0.780
560	0.22	22.0	0.785
577	0.22	21.0	0.787
585	0.22	20.5	0.790
633	0.27	18.7	0.820

the cooler location. Consequently, there is a temperature rise at the cooler location and a temperature decrease at the hotter location until they are both at the same temperature.

The rate at which the temperature changes depends on the thermal diffusivity of the tissue (a constant equal to the thermal conductivity divided by tissue density and heat capacity), the size of the temperature difference, and the distance between the two locations. This implies that the rate at which the temperature changes will itself also change with time. Obviously, within tissue there are an infinite number of locations each of which may be conducting heat to other locations and/or receiving heat from other locations.

For our infinitesimally small volume at a given location the rate of change of the temperature rise (or fall) is governed by the heat conduction plus the rate of volumetric heat production as explained above. These two rates can be incorporated into one equation, called the heat equation (see, for example, Chen[10]), and this equation provides the temporal and spatial distribution of

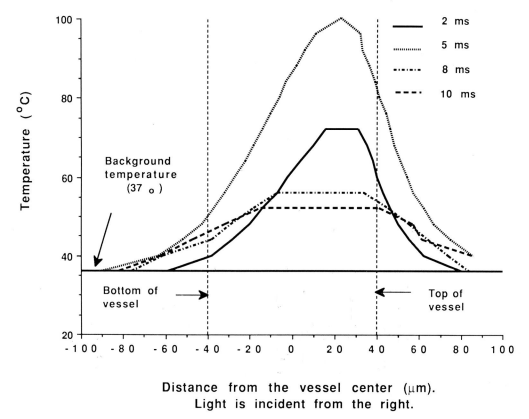

Fig. 2–5. The heating of an individual blood vessel. A 5 ms pulse of 410 W/cm² 577 nm light is incident on the top of an 80 μm diameter vessel (from the right). This figure shows the temperature of a section through the center of the vessel during the pulse (2 ms), at the end of the pulse (5 ms), and after the pulse (8, 10 ms). This combination of wavelength, fluence rate, and exposure time is sufficient to coagulate most of the blood within the vessel and to irreversibly damage the endothelial cells at the top of the vessel to a thickness of 5 to 10 μm (i.e., at the distance from the vessel center of 45–50 μm the maximum temperature is approximately 70° C).

the tissue temperature rise. Figure 2–5 illustrates the temperature distribution within and surrounding a blood vessel during and after a pulse of light incident on the top surface.

Tissue Damage. Finally, tissue damage is usually related to a combination of local temperature rise and the duration of that temperature rise through a first-order rate process (see, for example, van Gemert et al.,[4] pages 218 to 221). From such a "damage-integral" description, a simpler method has been derived by defining a "critical temperature": if tissue has been for a certain duration at the critical temperature that is associated with that duration, the tissue is (locally) considered irreversibly damaged. Figure 2–6 shows an example of such a "critical temperature" versus exposure time curve. For the analysis to follow, however, the actual values of the critical temperatures play an unimportant role.

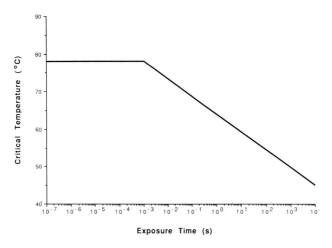

Fig. 2–6. The critical temperature for irreversible damage depends on the exposure time. For example, 70° C is required for 0.1 s exposure.[4]

Physics and Biologic Wound Healing

Figure 2–7 summarizes the key assumption of the modeling of PWS treated by a laser: a capillary is assumed: (a) to be irreversibly damaged; (b) to occlude; and (c) to have subsequent ideal wound healing (see Fig. 2–2), when the *top of the blood vessel* wall reaches the critical temperature during laser irradiation. An example is an assumed critical temperature of 70° C caused by a laser pulse of 0.1 s duration[2] (see also Fig. 2–6).

Laser–Port-Wine Stain Interactions

Short Exposure Times

Short exposure times are defined here according to Table 2–1: *long* enough to heat up the red blood cells, to conduct that heat from the red blood cells to the vessel wall and irreversibly damage the wall, but *short* enough to prevent irreversible damage to a substantial dermal tissue volume. Such exposure

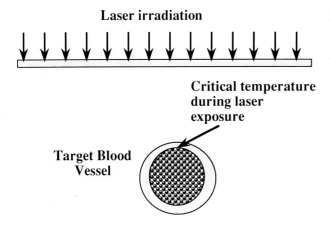

Fig. 2–7. The goal for our model, which we assume results in ideal wound healing (Fig. 2–2), is to attain the critical temperature at the top of the target blood vessel lumen.

Fig. 2–8. The absorption coefficients as a function of wavelength for dermis, epidermis (this may vary by a factor of two or more depending on the quantity of melanin within the epidermis), and oxygenated blood (hematocrit of 40).

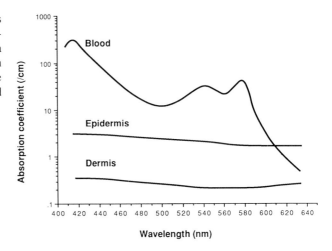

times are around 1 ms. It is noted that irradiation times shorter than about 0.1 ms lead to explosive vaporization of blood, to tearing of the ectatic capillary, to a biologic response that does not lead to occlusion of the capillary, and, hence, to an insufficient laser treatment of the stain.[11,12]

Under such circumstances of short exposure times, local tissue temperature rise can be assumed to be directly proportional to local heat production (because very little heat conduction occurs during the pulse) and, hence, to the product of local absorption coefficient and local fluence rate (Fig. 2–4).

Depth of Vascular Damage: The Best Wavelength

Figure 2–8 shows the absorption coefficients of whole blood (oxyhemoglobin, 40% hematocrit) and of epidermis and dermis as a function of wavelength. Table 2–3 shows the absorption coefficients, scattering coefficients, and anisotropy factors of scattering for these tissues at selected wavelengths. From these data, Figure 2–9 shows results from Monte Carlo computations of skin fluence rate distributions for several wavelengths,

Fig. 2–9. The fluence rate, relative to a 1 W/cm^2 (6 mm diameter) incident beam, through bloodless dermis for 415, 545, 577, and 585 nm. The absorption in the epidermis (Fig. 2–8 and Table 2–3) has the greatest influence in this case.

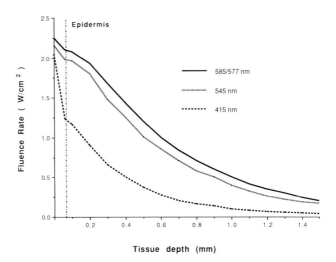

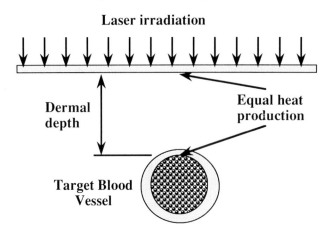

Laser irradiation

Dermal depth

Equal heat production

Target Blood Vessel

Fig. 2–10. The criterion for selective coagulation of blood vessels is that the heat production at the top of the target vessel lumen is no greater than that at the epidermis-dermis interface.

assuming a bloodless dermis. The heat production associated with 577 nm irradiation is shown in Figure 2–4.

Figure 2–10 indicates how the maximum depth of selective vascular damage can be inferred from Figure 2–9. The criterion is that the heat production at the epidermis-dermis interface equals the heat production at the top of the red blood cells in the capillary lumen. In other words, a dermal depth is sought at which the product of epidermal absorption coefficient (Table 2–3) and fluence rate at the epidermis-dermis junction (Fig. 2–9) equals the product of blood absorption coefficient (Table 2–3) and fluence rate at the dermis–blood vessel junction. This latter fluence rate (dermis–blood vessel junction) equals the dermal fluence rate (Fig. 2–9) because it is assumed for simplicity that the presence of a blood vessel does not influence the fluence rate distribution inside the dermis. There is no doubt that this assumption is an approximation, and Monte Carlo computations have to be used in the future to test the validity of this assumption and to improve on this part of the analysis.

Single-Vessel PWS Model: The Case for 577 nm?

Figure 2–11 shows the results of the above analysis, for the single-vessel PWS model of Figure 2–1A. The analysis predicts a maximum dermal depth of vascular damage of about 1.8 mm for the 577 nm yellow wavelength, but virtually the same value for the 415 nm violet wavelength(!). The argon laser blue-green wavelengths (488/515 nm) are predicted to have a selective dermal vascular depth of 0.85 mm, and the frequency-doubled Nd:YAG laser at 532 nm, of about 1.4 mm.

Because of our model assumption that a vessel is irreversibly damaged once the *top* of the vessel wall is damaged, it is intuitively clear that optimal wavelengths to treat a PWS coincide with maxima in the oxyhemoglobin curve. Hence, 577 nm is predicted to be a better wavelength than 585 nm.

Multi-Vessel PWS Model: The Case for 585 nm?

For the multi-vessel PWS model (Fig. 2–1B,C), Figure 2–3 holds the key to the possible explanation that 585 nm is a better wavelength for PWS treatment than 577 nm. The figure shows that for a constant irradiance the

Fig. 2–11. For the single-vessel model (bloodless dermis, Fig. 2–1a), the maximum depth to which a vessel can be selectively coagulated (the criteria of Fig. 2–10) as a function of the wavelength.

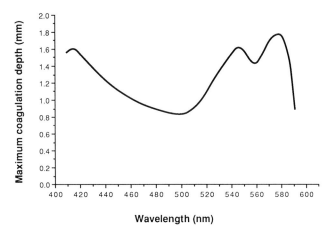

fluence rate spatial distribution inside the skin depends strongly upon the laser beam diameter.[9] Further, the tissue depth where the fluence rate reaches the target vessel's coagulation threshold depends upon the blood volume of vessels anterior to the target vessel. The anterior vessels absorb laser light before it reaches the target vessel. Thus, 577 nm, with the largest blood absorption in the yellow, penetrates less deeply than 585 nm (for an equal irradiance and spot diameter), and 585 nm penetrates less deeply than, say, 590 nm. Obviously, 415 nm with its extremely large blood absorption penetrates substantially less deeply than 577 nm.

Crucial for treatment of PWS is the amount of heat produced at the top of the vessel lumen; this must be adequate for irreversible damage of the whole vessel. The 577 nm wavelength has 1.85 times more absorption in blood than 585 nm, and 5.1 times more than 590 nm (blood absorption coefficients of, respectively, 35.4 mm^{-1} at 577 nm, 19.1 mm^{-1} at 585 nm, and 6.9 mm^{-1} at 590 nm). Using Figure 2–1C as the PWS model, and the criterion for selective vessel damage as explained in Figure 2–10, Monte Carlo computations yield the results shown in Figure 2–12. For a PWS with more than about 2% by volume of dermal blood, 585 nm produces deeper vascular damage than 577 nm, and 590 nm produces the least depth of vascular damage up until a 10% blood content of the stain. For PWS with more than 10% dermal blood content, however, our results suggest that 590 nm produces deeper vascular damage than 577 nm.[13]

Figure 2–12 clearly shows that, within the validity of our model assumptions, the ideal wavelength for PWS treatment depends upon the amount of dermal blood and hence on the PWS vascular anatomy. Our predictions do not match *quantitatively* the histologic data of Tan et al.,[3] who found selective vascular damage at 585 nm at a dermal depth of 1.2 mm, and at 577 nm of 0.72 mm. The model predicts, respectively, 0.70 mm and 0.56 mm with 5% blood by volume. The reason(s) for this quantitative discrepancy is (are) at present not understood, although, obviously, the uncertainty in the optical properties of the skin constituents and the resulting uncertainties in the predictions of the light fluence rate distributions play an important role. The question, however, remains whether we have overlooked an as yet unknown but important mechanism for producing irreversible vascular damage.

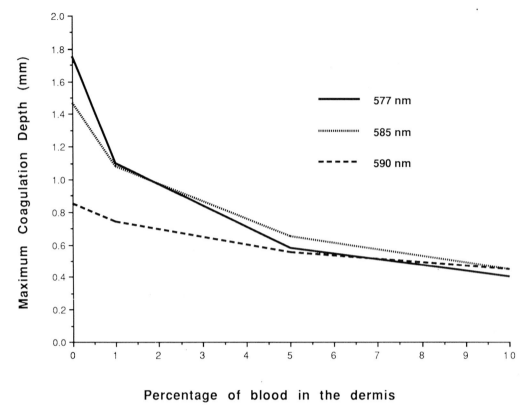

Fig. 2–12. For the blood filled dermis model (Fig. 2–1c), the maximum depth to which a vessel can be selectively coagulated (the criteria of Fig. 2–10) depends on both the wavelength and the quantity of blood within the dermis. For more than 1–2% blood within the dermis, 585 nm will produce a greater coagulation depth than 577 nm. At still greater quantities of blood (greater than 10%), 590 nm will produce the deepest coagulation.

Nevertheless, Figure 2–12 confirms Tan's result *qualitatively* in that 585 nm is a better wavelength than 577 nm or 590 nm to treat PWS. The reason for this is assumed to be the influence of the absorbing blood vessels on the depth of light penetration.

The Best Spot Diameter

Reports of the treatment of PWS with millisecond ($\sim$0.45 ms) yellow laser pulses refer to the total incident energy density (J/cm^2) as the key parameter that is to be related to the final clinical outcome. In other words, clinically, the conditions used for producing Figure 2–3 are obeyed: a constant incident irradiance (which is equal to the incident energy density in J/cm^2 divided by the exposure time) and a variable laser spot diameter. It is clear from Figure 2–3 that under such circumstances the spot diameter has to be in excess of 3 mm (for a wavelength around 580 nm) to produce the deepest fluence rate distribution inside the skin. The best spot diameter for PWS treatment is therefore at least 3 mm diameter.[9]

Longer Exposure Times

Longer exposure times imply that substantial heat conduction occurs from the "hot" structures such as epidermis and blood vessels to the "colder" structures such as the dermal collagen tissue, which has the lowest absorption coefficient for wavelengths below about 600 nm (see Fig. 2–8).

Heat Conduction from the Hot Epidermis. The *iron heater effect* refers to a hot epidermis that heats the underlying dermis through heat conduction, as if it were an iron heater. Figure 2–13 shows that an "epidermis" of 100° C temperature heats an equally thick layer of dermis (to a depth of, say, the same thickness as the epidermis, about 0.06 mm) to a temperature of 70° C within 0.023 seconds. Note, however, that in reality the epidermis is heated during laser irradiation, producing less iron heater effect than considered in Figure 2–13. A numerical analysis shows that 60 μm of dermis is irreversibly damaged after 0.01 s of (argon) laser irradiation (Fig. 15 of van Gemert et al.[4]), a shorter exposure time than is used clinically with the argon laser.

So, laser exposure times shorter than about 10 to 20 ms are required to prevent substantial dermal heating by heat conduction from the hot (100° C, say) epidermis.

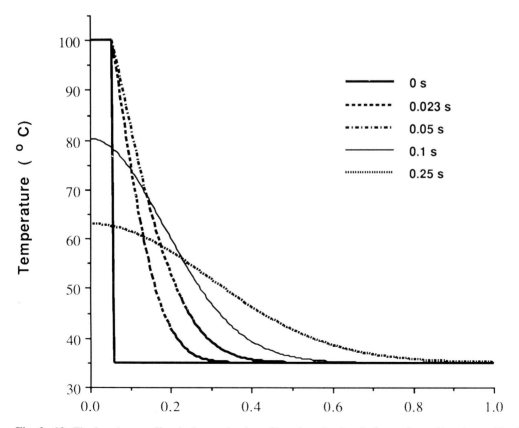

Fig. 2–13. The iron heater effect is the conduction of heat into the dermis from a hot epidermis resulting in nonspecific damage to a large volume of dermal tissue (and, therefore, possibly, contributes to scar formation). This is for a 60 μm thick epidermis maintained at a temperature of 100° C for 0.05 seconds.

Heat Conduction from Hot Blood Vessels. Figure 2–5 shows the situation of radial heat conduction from an irradiated "hot" vascular tube in dermal tissue. In previous work, Pickering et al.[14] have computed numerically the time required to heat cells at the top of the blood vessel to 70° C, from irradiation of the whole blood vessel by 578 nm. The results, summarized in Table 2–4, show that these exposure times are around 5 ms for vessels of about 0.1 mm diameter.

For larger-diameter blood vessels, and vessel wall thicknesses between 3 and 6 μm, a one-dimensional model becomes a reasonable approximation of the thermal response. Assuming a sudden temperature increase of the red blood cell lumen to 100° C, about 10^{-4} to 0.3×10^{-3} of heat conduction is required to heat the outer part of the wall to 70° C. Similarly, but now assuming that 80° C is required for the vessel wall cells to be irreversibly damaged, it requires between 0.2 ms (3 μm wall thickness) and 0.8 ms (6 μm wall thickness). These time durations lengthen, however, when heating of the lumen is considered.

In summary, depending upon the temperature conditions that are assumed, several milliseconds of heat conduction duration are ideally required to have the vessel wall coagulated transmurally. These conduction durations reduce to a few tenths of a millisecond, however, when the red blood cells are quickly heated (less than 10^{-4} s, say) to 100° C.

Speculations on the "Best" Laser Parameters for PWS Treatment

Despite the long tradition in laser treatment of PWS, which goes back to the early 1960s, the "best" laser parameters are still not assessable with certainty. According to Tan et al.,[3] the best wavelength is 585 nm and the best spotsize is 3 to 5 mm, with an incident energy density of 5 to 10 J/cm². The best exposure time is not so clearly specified, but has often been proposed as *shorter* than the "thermal relaxation time" of a capillary. This is around 3 ms for a 0.1 mm diameter vessel, and around 0.6 ms for a 0.05 mm diameter vessel.

Table 2–4. Results From Numerical Computations That Calculate the Required Incident Power Density on a Blood Vessel to Obtain 70° C Temperature at the Outer Side of the Vessel Wall*

	To coagulate the endothelial cells of 6 μm thickness requires:	
Vessel diameter (μm)	*Power density (W/cm²)*	*Exposure time (ms)*
15	2100	8.8
30	740	5.9
50	520	5.5
80	410	5.0
100	390	5.0

*Source: Pickering JW, Butler PH, Ring BJ, Walker EP. Computed temperature distributions around ectatic capillaries exposed to yellow (578 nm) laser light. Phys Med Biol 34:1–11, 1989

From a modeling standpoint we have to acknowledge that the results of modeling do not quantitatively agree with clinical histologic results. Therefore, it is only possible to give the *best speculations* for laser parameters at this time.

Wavelength. The best wavelength produces the deepest vascular damage with the least possible damage to the epidermal melanin. According to our model assumptions this wavelength is 577 nm, or larger rather than shorter because melanin absorbs less strongly at longer wavelengths. So, the wavelength of choice is between 577 and, say, 590 nm, with 585 nm most likely as a good compromise. For these reasons our model predicts, e.g., that 532 nm is less effective than the above wavelengths between 577 and 590 nm. However, our modeling also predicts this best wavelength to depend on the PWS vascular anatomy, in particular the dermal blood content, and the laser beam diameter.

Spot Diameter. In view of the penetrating properties of light, relative to incident irradiance, the best spot diameter is larger than 3 mm. This is clearly shown in Figure 2–3, and is in accordance with animal experimental results by Tan et al.[15]

Exposure Time. The exposure time should be sufficiently long to conduct heat from the hot red blood cell filled lumen to the outer part of the vessel wall. For a wall thickness between 3 and 6 μm, assuming the lumen to be 100° C during irradiation, and assuming 70° C is adequate for irreversible wall damage, the model predicts exposure times between 0.1 and 0.3 ms. Numerical computations by Pickering et al.[14] show that exposure times of about 5 ms are required to heat up the outer part of the wall to 70° C.

One of the unknowns in this sort of analysis is the absorption coefficient of the capillary wall itself, and hence the wall temperature rise caused by direct absorption of the laser light. When the absorption coefficient for bloodless dermal tissue is used (0.22 mm^{-1}), the heat conduction equation predicts a temperature rise of this wall, caused by a 10 J/cm^2 fluence, of about 6 to 7° C. However, absorption coefficients of normal human cadaver aorta, measured by Keijzer et al.[8] as 0.5 mm^{-1} to 1.2 mm^{-1}, yield a temperature rise of 14 to 34° C. In these latter situations, the *additional* temperature rise required for coagulation is produced by heat conduction in a shorter time than predicted above.

Irradiation should not tear the vessel wall, as this has been shown to be inefficient for blanching of the PWS; thus the pulse duration should be longer than 0.1 ms.

Hence, according to our best speculations the irradiation time should be longer than 0.1 ms and shorter than 10 ms.

Modeling the Color Appearance of PWS

The main morbidity of a PWS is its excessive red color appearance. Despite the importance of color in the treatment of PWS, very little is known about the contribution of dermal capillaries to the color appearance of the stain. Such information would obviously contribute to the knowledge of the required depth of irreversible vascular damage. In the early 1980s, Finley et al.[16] [1981] stated that the ectatic vessels require irreversible damage down to a dermal depth of at least 0.5 mm. Recently, Tan et al.[3] [1990] showed in 6 patients that dermal depth greater than 1 mm for irreversible vascular damage is a more likely requirement to compensate fully for the excess red color of the stain.

The color appearance of an object relates to the spectral concentration of radiance that is remitted from that object. By knowing this spectral remittance in response to an appropriate incident spectral distribution (like "day light"), and by comparing it with the eye's spectral sensitivity curve, the color appearance occurs through three primary colors (red, green, and blue). The appearance of the object is used to classify that color in a three-dimensional color-space.

This is the field of the science of color, a part of physics that is highly technical and that we cannot explain in detail here. We refer in the literature to the book by Wyszecki and Stiles for details.[17]

In this paragraph we present results of preliminary attempts to model the color difference between a "treated" and an "untreated" PWS. Figure 2–14 shows the *untreated* PWS. It consists of an epidermis of thickness 0.06 mm with absorbing and scattering properties as a function of wavelength according to Table 2–3. The dermis extends infinitely deep and is also characterized optically according to the data of Table 2–3. The dermis has an amount of ectatic blood vessels that is assumed to occupy 5 or 10% of the dermal volume.[5] Blood is optically characterized by the data in Figure 2–8 and Table 2–3. The *treated* PWS involves the same epidermis as the untreated stain. The dermis, however, is divided into a layer that involves no blood (the *treated* dermal depth, identical in its optical properties to healthy skin) and the remaining dermal layer, which still involves the 5 or 10% blood content. In the model, healthy skin consists of epidermis and dermis with optical properties summarized in Table 2–3 and with a blood content of 0%.

Remittance as a function of wavelength is calculated by using the diffusion approximation to the transport equation in one dimension, assuming that skin has a refractive index of 1.37. These computations have been performed for wavelengths of 415, 500, 540, 560, 577, and 633 nm. The color appearance of the PWS, as a function of "treatment-depth" is then calculated. Finally, the *color difference* (Delta E) between treated PWS and healthy skin is assessed according to formulae given in Wyszecki and Stiles [ref.17, Eqs. 5(3.3.9), page 167]. This color difference is the distance between two points in three-dimensional color-space that represent, respectively, the partly-treated PWS and healthy skin colors.

It is not easy to define a criterion for Delta E where color matching between treated PWS and healthy skin has occurred to a reasonable degree (in view of changes in skin color owing to, e.g., environmental changes such as cold, warm, blush, etc.). We have chosen a threshold value of

$$Delta\ E = 0.5$$

which was obtained by visually comparing the predicted colors that were produced on a color screen.

Fig. 2–14. (a) For color quantification of port-wine stains we have assumed the lesions consist of blood homogeneously spread through the dermis with 5 to 10% by volume. (b) The ectatic vessels contributing to this blood volume tend to be treated from the top of the dermis down, and we have assumed that during treatment there is a certain depth at which there is essentially no additional blood. (c) Eventually, normal-looking (healthy) skin results in which any remaining ectatic capillaries are at such a great depth that they no longer contribute to the skin color.

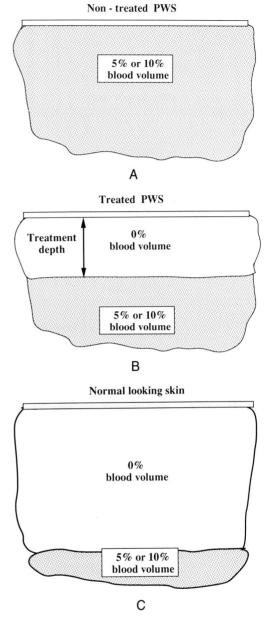

The results are shown in Figure 2–15. They show that color matching of a PWS defined in Figure 2–14 is virtually complete when ectatic vessels are irreversibly damaged down to a dermal depth of about 0.9 to 1.0 mm, in good agreement with the histologic observations of Tan et al.[3]

Discussion and Conclusions

Laser treatment of PWS is one of the few clinical procedures in which modeling resulted in an improved treatment strategy: from the blue-green argon laser, at 0.2 s irradiation and a 1 mm spot size, to the yellow flashlamp

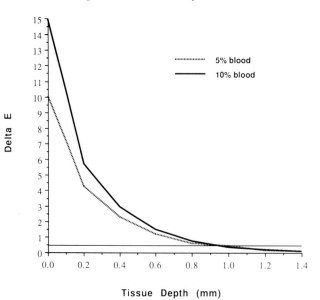

Fig. 2–15. Our color model suggests that below a ΔE-value of 0.5 there is no difference between skin absent of ectatic vessels and PWS skin in which the ectatic vessels below a certain depth contribute 5 or 10% by volume.

Tissue Depth (mm)

pumped dye laser at 577 nm, 0.45 ms, and 3 to 5 mm spot size. The next step of improvement, from 577 to 585 nm, under otherwise identical conditions of irradiation time (0.45 ms) and spot size (3 to 5 mm), occurred in the usual way: from clinical intuition via animal experiments[18] to clinical justification.[3]

The physical mechanism that might be responsible for the observation that a wavelength of 585 nm produces deeper vascular injury than one of 577 nm has been explained in this chapter. It is proposed that light scattering in skin, combined with an increase in (overall) dermal absorption owing to the blood content of the ectatic capillaries, causes 585 nm to penetrate and damage vascular structures at a deeper dermal level than 577 nm or 590 nm. It is important to note that the criterion that translates physics into biologic wound healing plays an important role in the assessment of the "best" wavelength. In this chapter it is proposed that irreversible damage of the top of the blood vessel wall produces occlusion of the whole vessel with subsequent "ideal" wound healing of the skin. This criterion has been used previously to explain that 577 nm is a much better wavelength to treat PWS than 488/515 nm of an argon laser. We emphasize, however, that it is currently unknown to what degree this criterion is valid, if at all. So far, we are lacking a clear hemodynamic criterion to explain under what physical constraints a capillary will thrombose.

Despite these uncertainties in the modeling assumptions, it is interesting to discuss the possible consequences of our model. First, it predicts that the best wavelength for PWS treatment depends upon the PWS anatomy itself—in particular, upon the amount of dermal volumetric blood. Second, the best wavelength deviates from 577 nm when many dermal blood capillaries are irradiated by the laser beam. For very small laser beams, therefore, the deviation from 577 nm is expected to disappear. For longer irradiation times heat conduction will enlarge the dermal volume around a "hot" capillary, and it seems reasonable to expect that, under those conditions, the difference in clinical response between 577 and 585 nm will tend to disappear. So it is predicted that for CW dye lasers there will be virtually no difference in clinical outcome between 577 and 585 nm.

As discussed in our introductory paragraphs, the criteria relating physical parameters (such as temperature rise) to the skin's biologic response is critical to the modeling. The calculations for the irreversible damage to the vessel do not take into account the target vessel size.

If we take as an alternative criterion for vessel damage that the *center* rather than the top of the vessel rise to the critical temperature, then in general the conclusions of our laser–PWS interactions analysis and Figure 2–12 apply. However, there is now an additional vessel size dependence which illustrates that the larger the vessels the greater the difference in maximum coagulation depth between 585 and 577 nm (Fig. 2–16).

For very large vessels (>150 µm diameter), 590 nm can be used effectively. The penetration in blood of 590 nm light is so great that for smaller vessels too high a percentage of light penetrates the whole vessel without being absorbed, and thus the temperature rise is insufficient to damage the vessels. It is also noteworthy that this new criterion reduces the maximum coagulation depth for all wavelengths and has the minimum coagulation depth for the maximum vessel sizes.

The depths of irreversible vascular damage predicted by our models and those observed histologically by Tan et al.[3] disagree by a factor of about two. This discrepancy is not well understood, although uncertainties in the optical properties of skin tissues suggest the "easiest" possibility. Indeed, current evidence has been found that especially absorption coefficients measured by integrating sphere methods may be too large.[19] It is, however, too early to

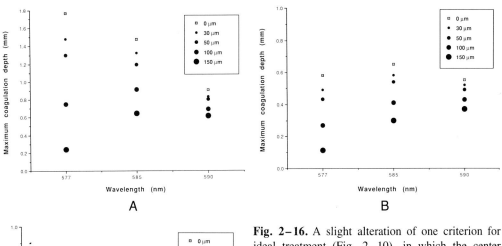

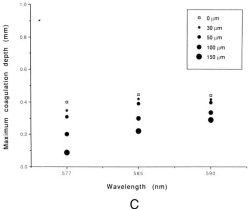

Fig. 2–16. A slight alteration of one criterion for ideal treatment (Fig. 2–10), in which the center rather than the top of the vessel lumen is to reach the critical temperature, results in an overall lowering of the dermal coagulation depth, but also a vessel size dependence. (a) 0% blood dermis. (b) 5% blood dermis. (c) 10% blood dermis.

comment on this here. Based upon the present modeling results, we cannot exclude that there is an as yet unknown mechanism that contributes to producing irreversible vascular injury.

The criterion for the "best" exposure time is irreversible damage of the vascular wall by way of heat conduction from the heated red blood cells in the lumen of the vessel. Despite the fact that this is a clear criterion, it does not clearly define a "best" exposure time. Numerical computations of heat conduction suggest "a few" milliseconds, but simplified conduction estimates suggest that a few tenths of a millisecond may be adequate. As a result, we can only say that the exposure time should be longer than the 0.1 ms that is known to produce tearing of the vessel wall,[12] and shorter than 10 ms that will produce too much dermal injury by heat conduction.

The criterion for the "best" spot diameter is that diameter which produces the maximum fluence rate penetration depth per incident irradiance. Because of the strong scattering properties of the skin layers, this turns out to be a laser beam diameter of at least 3 mm.

Appendix: Terminology

For the following discussion of terminology we have attempted to adhere to the standards as defined by Sliney.[20]

Light may be considered as particles (photons) or electromagnetic waves. As a wave, light is defined in terms of its *wavelength* in *nanometers* (nm; 1 nm = 10^{-9} of a meter). We recognize visible light of different wavelengths as different colors. If we consider light in terms of photons (all traveling at a constant speed, i.e., the speed of light), then for each wavelength all the photons have an identical energy, unique to that wavelength. Energy is normally quantified in units of *Joules* (J). The combination of the energy of the photons and the rate at which they arrive at a given location (i.e., number of photons per unit time multiplied by the photon energy) is the *power* (J/s; or Watts, W).

Light is incident on the skin over a finite area (the spot size in cm²). The total energy incident per unit area (J/cm²) has been often referred to as the *surface exposure dose* or just the *dose* in photobiology. As dose is defined differently in radiometric terms, the term *radiant exposure* may be used instead to avoid confusion. Note that the radiant exposure is often referred to as *energy density;* similarly, the power per unit area (W/cm²) as the *power density*. However, standard radiometric terminology reserves these terms for the energy and power per unit volume rather than per unit area. The incident power per unit area is most commonly called the *irradiance*.

Within the tissue the photons are no longer confined to the two dimensions (traveling in approximately the same direction as they are incident on the skin), but are scattered in random directions. To describe the distribution of light within the tissue the terms *fluence* (J/cm²) and *fluence rate* (W/cm²) are used. Rigorously, the fluence is the number of photons, multiplied by their energy, that are incident on a small sphere within the tissue, divided by the cross-sectional area of that sphere. And the fluence rate is defined as the fluence per unit time.

As the photons pass through a certain point within the tissue, there is a certain probability that they will be absorbed; this leads to heat production. The rate at which the photons are absorbed depends on the product of the fluence rate and an *absorption coefficient* (/cm), and may be described as the rate at which energy is deposited per unit volume (W/cm^3); for simplicity we may refer to this as the *deposition rate*.

References

1. Mordon S, Rotteleur G, Buys B, Brunetaud JM. Comparative study on the "point by point" technique and the "scanning" technique for laser treatment of the port-wine stains. Lasers Surg Med 9:398, 1989.
2. Gemert MJC van, Kleijn WJ de, Hulsbergen-Henning JP. Temperature behaviour of a model port-wine stain during argon laser coagulation. Phys Med Biol 27:1089, 1982.
3. Tan OT, Morrison P, Kurban AK. 585 nm for the treatment of portwine stains. Plast Reconstr Surg 86:1112, 1990.
4. Gemert MJC van, Welch AJ, Miller ID, Tan OT. Can physical modeling lead to an optimal laser treatment strategy for port-wine stains? *In* Wolbarsht ML (ed). Laser Applications in Medicine and Biology, Vol 5. New York, Plenum Press, 1991, p 199.
5. Barsky SH, Rosen S, Geer DE, Noe JM. The nature and evolution of port wine stains: A computer assisted study. J Invest Dermatol 74:154, 1980.
6. Anderson RR, Parrish JA. Microvasculature can be selectively damaged using dye lasers: A basic theory and experimental evidence in human skin. Lasers Surg Med 1:263, 1981.
7. Gemert MJC van, Hulsbergen-Henning JP. A model approach to laser coagulation of dermal vascular lesions. Arch Dermatol Res 270:429, 1981.
8. Keijzer M, Jacques SL, Prahl SA, Welch AJ. Light distributions in artery tissue: Monte Carlo simulations for finite-diameter laser beams. Lasers Surg Med 9:148, 1989.
9. Keijzer M, Pickering BW, van Gemert MJC. Laser beam diameter for portwine stain treatment. Lasers Surg Med in press 1991.
10. Chen MM. The tissue energy balance equation. In: A Shitzer, RC Eberhart (Eds), Heat transfer in medicine and biology. p 153, Plenum Press, New York, 1985.
11. Hulsbergen-Henning JP, Gemert MJC van, Lahaye CTW. Clinical and histological evaluation of portwine stain treatment with a microsecond-pulsed dye laser at 577 nm. Lasers Surg Med 4:375, 1984.
12. Garden JM, Tan OT, Kerschmann R et al. Effect of dye laser pulse duration on selective cutaneous vascular injury. J Invest Dermatol 87:653, 1986.
13. Pickering BW, van Gemert MJC. 585 nm for the laser treatment of port wine stains: A possible mechanism. Lasers Surg Med in press 1991.
14. Pickering JW, Butler PH, Ring BJ, Walker EP. Computed temperature distributions around ectatic capillaries exposed to yellow (578 nm) laser light. Phys Med Biol 34:1247, 1989.
15. Tan OT, Motamedi M, Welch AJ, Kurban AK. Spotsize effects on guinea pig skin following pulsed irradiation. J Invest Dermatol 90:877, 1988.
16. Finley JL, Barsky SH, Geer DE. Healing of portwine stains after argon laser therapy. Arch Dermatol 117:486, 1981.
17. Wyszecki G, Stiles WS. Color Science: Concepts and Methods, Quantitative Data and Formulae. 2nd Ed. New York, Wiley, 1982.
18. Tan OT, Murray S, Kurban AK. Action spectrum of vascular specific injury using pulsed irradiation. J Invest Dermatol 92:868, 1989.
19. Torres JH. Thermal response of arterial wall to continuous wave laser irradiation and contact probe application. PhD Thesis, The University of Texas at Austin, 1991, p 75.
20. Sliney DH. Dosimetric concepts for optical radiation. SPIE Institute Series, Vol 155, p 16, 1989.

Chapter 3   Evaluation, Diagnosis, and Selection of Patients for Laser and Nonlaser Treatment

Amal K. Kurban

Lasers are characterized by coherent, monochromatic light of high intensity. Their action depends on the absorption of this energy by a chromophore where the light energy is converted into heat that injures or destroys tissue. Hemoglobin is one of the two most common, naturally occurring chromophores in the skin. Hence, all skin lesions comprised of channels filled with hemoglobin-containing erythrocytes are potential targets for lasers and could be laser-treated. The selection of patients with vascular disorders for laser treatment depends on the diagnosis and overall evaluation of such patients.

The classification of cutaneous vascular lesions is complicated. In Chapter 1, Dr. Mulliken outlined the principles that form the basis for a workable classification. Some of these conditions are best treated by laser (e.g., port-wine stain); others could be treated by laser as well as other modalities (e.g., pyogenic granuloma); and still others are best treated by nonlaser methods (e.g., arborizing telangiectasia of the legs). As a result, an accurate diagnosis is essential for a favorable therapeutic outcome.

Components of Evaluation

When a patient with a cutaneous vascular lesion consults a physician, the evaluation should consist of a detailed history, complete physical examination, and selected laboratory tests.

Detailed History. The medical history (see Table 3–1) should include not only details of the vascular lesion itself, but also information concerning the patient's general health, including any history of bleeding, seizures, or eye problems. Account should also be taken of current and previous medications, allergies, the patient's occupation, social habits, and hobbies, and family history of similar lesions.

Questions pertaining to the vascular lesion itself should include these areas of detail:

1. *Age of onset.* Even though port-wine stains and hemangiomas are "present since birth," the former are characteristically so, whereas hemangiomas appear at a later age. Hereditary hemorrhagic telangiectasia appears from the second decade onward; facial telangiectasias, with or without rosacea, and senile angiomas tend to appear from the fourth decade onward. Spider angiomas often appear with pregnancy or with cirrhosis of the liver.

2. *Evolution of the lesion.* Hemangiomas characteristically go through a growing phase followed by regression. Port-wine stains are notoriously stable, and their growth is commensurate with that of the body. Salmon patches, on the other hand, involute completely, and 30 to 50% of the nuchal lesions disappear.

3. *History of bleeding, ulceration, infection.* These are complications not infrequently seen in hemangiomas and may be an indication for instituting treatment. Similarly, patients with hereditary hemorrhagic telangiectasia (Rendu-Osler-Weber syndrome) present because of epistaxis or gastrointestinal bleeding.

4. *Change in size and color.* "Maturity" of a vascular lesion (like port-wine stain) is used to describe the darkening in color, increase in size, and the appearance of nodularities in an otherwise macular lesion.

5. *Associated pain and discomfort.* This is not unusual in patients with varicosities or even telangiectasias of the legs.

6. *Previous treatment.* This is important whether the treatment was for the vascular lesion or not. The usual treatment modalities for vascular lesions have been radiotherapy, electrodesiccation, tattooing, laser, sclerotherapy, and intralesional corticosteroids. The outcome of these treatment modalities and the resultant pigmentary changes and scarring may affect future treatment. A variety of medications may also adversely affect laser treatment, e.g., anticoagulants, vasodilators, aspirin. Since the laser would disrupt cutaneous vascular channels, any additive insult (dilatation or hemorrhage) might lead to hemorrhage

Table 3–1. Details of Vascular Lesion by History

- Age of onset
- Evolution of lesion
- Bleeding, ulceration, infection
- Change in size, color
- Associated symptoms
- Previous treatment
- Other findings

Table 3–2. Details of Vascular Lesion by Examination

Distribution	Localized or generalized Single or multiple Central or peripheral Dermatomal: which
Consistency	Macular or raised Uniformity of lesion Compressible or blanchable
Color	Shade of redness: pink, red, dark red, violet, dark blue
Vascularity	Individual vascular channels identifiable or matter Size of channels and depth
Extracutaneous involvement	Adjoining mucosa and conjunctiva Underlying soft-tissue hypertrophy
Associated findings	

(with resultant hemosiderin deposition), necrosis, infection, and scarring.

7. *Other findings*. History of seizures and eye problems is important, especially if any is associated with a port-wine stain involving the trigeminal dermatome. There is evidence that bilateral distribution of the birthmark, involvement of both upper and lower eyelids, and unilateral involvement of areas served by the three branches of the trigeminal nerve are associated with a significantly higher incidence of central nervous system (seizures) and/or eye (glaucoma) complications.[1] Similarly, some neurocutaneous syndromes encompass a cutaneous vascular lesion and concomitant neural involvement. There is increasing evidence that some of the vascular lesions have a genetic background.

Physical Examination. The examination should encompass complete evaluation of the skin surface (color and type of skin should be noted) and of the oral mucosa. The location, distribution, and size of the vascular lesions should be noted, preferably through use of a diagram. For a detailed examination, see Table 3–2.

Laboratory Tests. Tests may be needed to determine whether there is anemia, tendency toward bleeding, or any other underlying disorder (e.g., connective tissue disease, liver cirrhosis). In obscure cases a physician will resort to a skin biopsy to ensure a proper evaluation and diagnosis of the condition. Consultation with other specialists, such as ophthalmologists or neurologists, may be needed.

Treatment Method and Selection Criteria

Aided by the above, the physician can arrive at a diagnosis and determine whether the vascular lesion is amenable to treatment, and whether the treatment should be laser or nonlaser.

Nonlaser treatment is recommended for the hemangioma group of lesions, which ordinarily regress spontaneously, except in specific instances where the hemangioma could affect the function of a vital organ (e.g., eye) or is subject to ulceration and secondary infection (see Chapter 10). In these instances laser treatment then may induce a regression phase. Laser treatment is also indicated for any remaining vascular channels after a hemangioma has regressed. Nonlaser treatment is further recommended for "arborizing telangiectasias" of the lower extremities (2), as well as for varicosities of the legs (see Chapter 13). To date, laser treatment in these areas has been disappointing.[2]

Laser treatment is recommended for all other benign cutaneous vascular lesions; among these are port-wine stains as well as primary and secondary telangiectasia. Further selection for laser treatment takes into account several "host" factors: age, skin type, and previous treatment of the vascular lesion.

Age. It has been amply demonstrated that the earlier port-wine stains are treated, the better the results.[3] Previous experience with nonpulsed lasers (e.g., CO_2, Argon) resulted in a high incidence of scarring, most often in children under the age of 18 years.[4] With the advent of pulsed lasers, however, by which the pulse duration, fluence, and wavelength are controlled, the incidence of scarring has been negligible, and the results of treatment on children have been very gratifying. Hence, it is recommended that treatment be started as soon as possible, underscoring the advantages of such a policy: the size of the vascular lesion is relatively small; there is minimal or no tissue hypertrophy in the affected area; treatment can be concluded before the age at which the child may be subjected to social and psychological trauma.

Skin Type (see Table 3–3). Melanin, the other main, naturally occurring cutaneous chromophore, is present in the epidermis. The pigment is elaborated by melanocytes present in the basal cell layer, and is then transferred to the keratinocytes. Melanin has a wide absorption spectrum. Anatomically, being in the epidermis, it acts as the first target for the laser beam. Thus, it stands to reason that the more pigment present in the epidermis, the greater the absorption of the laser energy by that layer, and consequently less energy is available to reach the blood vessels in the dermis. These theoretical conclusions have been confirmed experimentally.[5] Hence, in patients with Type VI skin, laser treatment of vascular lesions is not

Table 3–3. Classification of Skin Types According to History of Response to Sun Exposure

Type	Characteristics
I	Always burn, never tan
II	Always burn, tan less than average (with difficulty)
III	Sometimes would burn, tan average
IV	Rarely burn, tan more than average (with ease)
V	Moderately pigmented
VI	Black

indicated because very little energy reaches the vessels, and the concentration of the absorption by the epidermis could result in scarring, hypopigmentation, or hyperpigmentation. Patients with skin Types I to IV can be successfully treated with lasers, whereas those with Type V will have questionable outcome. The corollary to this is that patients with skin Types II to IV should be advised to stay out of the sun and use sunscreens because tanning could increase the pigmentation of the epidermis to the extent that a relatively greater portion of the laser beam is absorbed there. Consequently, dark-tanned patients are usually excluded from laser treatment until the tan has faded.

Previous Laser Treatment to the Vascular Lesion. Patients who have had unsuccessful laser treatment usually end up with scar formation as well as hyperpigmentation and hypopigmentation. Such patients seeking further laser treatment face the potential of unmasking more of the pigmentary abnormalities once the remnants of the vascular lesion are further reduced. There is evidence, however, that pulsed laser treatment would enhance the lightening of the port-wine stain and may even improve the surface pattern of the scar.[6]

Previous Treatment with Tattoos. The deposition of a dye to mask a cutaneous vascular lesion may be an obstacle to laser treatment. The dye may act as an exogenous chromogen and compete with the hemoglobin-containing erythrocytes, thereby decreasing the ability of the laser to ablate the abnormally dilated vessels. Furthermore, when the accessible vessels are ablated, the pigment of the tattoo remains, so that the tattooed area continues to appear ''different'' from the rest of the skin.

Our experience has been that treatment of areas that have already been treated using other modalities necessitates a higher laser fluence, and the outcome often still remains unsatisfactory.

Use of Anesthesia. With the use of the pulsed laser, the series of pulses is of exceedingly short duration. The impact of this on the skin does result in discomfort, often described as akin to the snapping of a hot rubber band. Adult patients can tolerate this sensation, and no anesthetic is needed. In children, however, especially those between the ages of 3 and 12 years, some sort of anesthetic is needed (for details, see Chapter 5).

References

1. Tallman B, Tan OT, Morelli JG, et al. Location of port-wine stains and the likelihood of ophthalmic and/or nervous system complications. Pediatrics 87:323, 1991.
2. Tan OT, Kurban AK. Laser treatment for arborizing telangiectasia. Perspectives in Plast Surg 4:171, 1990.
3. Tan OT, Sherwood K, Gilchrest BA. Treatment of children with port-wine stains using the flashlamp-pulsed tunable dye laser. N Engl J Med 320:416, 1989.
4. Dixon JA, Huether S, Rotering RH. Hypertrophic scarring in Argon laser treatment of port-wine stains. Plast Reconstr Surg 73:771, 1984.
5. Tan OT, Kerschmann R, Parrish JA. The effect of epidermal pigmentation on selective, vascular effects of pulsed laser. Lasers Surg Med 4:365, 1984.
6. Alster TS, Kurban AK, Grove GL, et al. Alteration of argon laser-induced scars by the pulsed dye laser.

Chapter 4 The Argon Laser in the Treatment of the Port-Wine Stain Birthmark[*]

John A.S. Carruth, Martin J.C. van Gemert, Peter G. Shakespeare

The argon laser was hailed as "a new ray of hope for portwine stains" in an editorial in *The Lancet* in 1981. Although some excellent results have been achieved with this laser, its limitations have been established over the past decade. It now seems possible that it may not yet have achieved its full potential.

Until the advent of the argon laser, the port-wine stain (PWS) was considered to be "essentially untreatable." Patients were usually told that no treatment was available and were simply advised to use makeup to conceal the birthmark. It has been estimated, however, that only one-third of patients use special makeup to cover the port-wine stain, and many of those who do use makeup are distressed to be seen by others without this protection.

Treatment techniques in the past have included the most inappropriate applications of radiation, either by external radiotherapy or the application of thorium X or radioactive phosphorus. At best this appeared to have had no particular benefits, and at worst—at least in part—these applications may have been responsible for the malignant skin changes which authors have seen in previously radiated port-wine stains. Other treatments have included dermabrasion, cryotherapy, overtattooing of the mark with opaque pigments, and excision of the involved skin with grafting. But none of these techniques has given consistently satisfactory results.

The development of lasers has provided a potential method for the treatment of port-wine stains. Particularly the argon, tuneable dye, copper vapor, and frequency-doubled Nd:YAG emit light of a suitable color and intensity that has the potential to damage the blood vessels forming the birthmark without necessarily damaging the surrounding tissues. The laser most widely used to date is the argon laser, which produces blue/green light at a number of wavelengths, 80% of it at 488 and 515 nm. This light can be transmitted through clear and colorless structures without absorption and,

[*]The authors gratefully acknowledge permission of Dr. J. Pieter Hulsbergen-Henning (Veldhoven, The Netherlands) to quote some of his clinical results prior to publication, and discussions with Dr. John W. Pickering on the content of the manuscript.

therefore, without causing thermal damage. It is, however, absorbed by pigmented and blood-containing tissues, resulting in a temperature rise of these tissues.

The early theoretic basis of argon-laser treatment was that the beam will pass through the clear, normal epidermis which overlies the port-wine stain and then be selectively absorbed by the blood in the abnormal capillary network in the outer dermis, causing thermal damage to the endothelium of these vessels, and hence thrombosis. Clinically, this coagulation is seen as blanching. Over a period of months the thrombosed vessel layer is replaced by colorless fibrous tissue with a marked reduction in the color of the birthmark. Following treatment, the epidermis should return to normal. If there are some areas of irreversibly damaged epidermis, it has always been considered that there is sparing of the secondary skin appendages from which essentially normal epidermis will regenerate.

Contrary to these assumptions, histologic examinations by Apfelberg et al.,[1] Finley et al.,[2] and Dixon et al.[3] showed general coagulation necrosis of the entire epidermis with injury to the papillary dermis, thrombosis of ectatic port-wine vessels, and preservation of dermal appendages. Observations 6 months after treatment showed obliteration of the previously noted port-wine stain vessels with reconstruction of the epidermis and fibrosis of the upper dermis. From this it can be shown that, although there is thrombosis of the pathologic vessels, there is also extensive nonspecific damage to the surrounding epidermis and dermis. Recently, Brauner et al.[4] stated that argon laser therapy produces a second-degree burn involving the upper one millimeter of epidermis and dermis. This burn may heal with not only a histologic scar, but also a clinically unsightly hypertrophic scar. Possibly the fibrosis in the upper dermis, which has been defined as a histologic scar, may play a significant role in the color perception of vessels deeper than this fibrotic layer.

The difference between the above-mentioned ''theoretic basis'' and histologic observations is well understood, and it is explained by van Gemert et al. in Chapter 2 of this book. The main reason is that the argon laser techniques that were clinically used all employed a low power (usually between 1 and 4 W). As a result of the low power, the irradiation time is of necessity much longer than the ''ideal irradiation time'' of 1 to 10 ms; hence the damage is not confined to the vasculature. Also, the blue/green argon laser wavelengths are considered ''less selective'' than the yellow (577 to 585 nm) wavelengths.

Two major problems make the final assessment of the value of the Argon laser difficult. First, no accepted ''optimal technique'' exists for the treatment of port-wine stains with this laser, and to date no study has been performed using parameters that are in any way close to the ''ideal parameters'' that have been defined in the previous paragraph.

A vast range of techniques has been described in the literature, and almost all give approximately the same results from the point of view of clearance of the birthmark and incidence of scarring. It must be stated, however, that all the techniques described to date use a laser-tissue interaction time that is several orders of magnitude greater than the ideal. It is not surprising, therefore, that similar clinical results are produced.

The second problem is that the reporting of results lacks objectivity, making it difficult to compare the results of the various series. Attempts have been made to report results objectively using color meters, reflectance spectrophotometry, or transcutaneous microscopy, but the quality of the results reported using these techniques does not always correlate with the final clinical results. A majority of authors make every effort to ensure that the clinical results which they report are as precise as possible, often using more than one observer; but it still remains extremely difficult, if not impossible, to compare results accurately. Quaba[5] has a composite scoring system using color, makeup, texture, and scarring as the features which are scored individually; total scores are then graded, as in almost all the other series, as excellent, good, fair, poor, and unacceptable. In his paper, Quaba indicates that other workers use as the definition of an excellent result "total blanching without scarring," "identical to normal skin," "virtually total blanching without scarring," and "virtually removed." Although one must always seek to report objective, and therefore comparable, results, it must be stressed again that objective results do not always correlate with the final clinical picture.

Time and carefully constructed studies will determine whether there is an ideal and optimal treatment technique for port-wine stain birthmarks, and whether the argon laser can produce parameters that are sufficiently close to these ideal parameters. A variety of techniques should be compared on the same patient. Research into treatment for PWS birthmarks has been severely hampered by the lack of any suitable animal model. Although the hen crest has been proposed for that purpose, significant differences do exist between the vessels in the hen crest and those in a port-wine stain birthmark.

It is of course vital, and has been stressed from the very early days of the argon laser, that all treatment parameters be fully recorded.[6] This must be combined with objective reporting of results in order that techniques and results from various centers can be compared accurately. Nonetheless, even with the most commonly used hand-held free-hand techniques, it is difficult to measure accurately the treatment parameters that must, of necessity, vary significantly. Some "computerized automatic techniques" have now been introduced by which treatment parameters can be set accurately; these will undoubtedly add to the establishment of an ideal technique—if, indeed, such a technique exists for all forms of birthmark in all patients.

Treatment Program

Consultation

The patient will normally be referred to the laser clinic by his or her family practitioner. It must be stated that there is considerable misunderstanding of the role of lasers in medicine and surgery, not just among the lay public, but also among the medical profession. The patient may therefore have a totally unrealistic expectation of the results which can be obtained with the argon-laser treatment of a port-wine stain. We believe that the first consultation should be with a doctor who is in a position to assess the patient's birthmark, to explain clearly the treatment program—and in particular its time scale—and to give a realistic assessment of the likely outcome, from the point of view both of the chance of a favorable result and of the chance of scarring. The doctor must clearly explain the limitations of the end point of the treatment technique, and he must indicate with clinical photographs if possible the types of scarring, namely atrophic and hypertrophic, which can occur. In this way the patient would be in a position to sign a "fully informed consent form." Details of all the information given to the patient must be clearly recorded, as, even in countries where litigation is not common, it may be vitally important to show in law exactly what had been said to the patient and what the patient had been told to expect.

Patient Selection

This remains extremely difficult. In the early stages of the development of the Argon laser every patient was accepted for treatment, as there was no method available for predicting those who would obtain a satisfactory result. Over the past decade, however, there has been increasing evidence that the argon laser is only of significant value for the treatment of "mature birthmarks," which naturally tend to occur in older patients, although occasionally they are found in a younger age group. In a review of the literature, Hobby stated that "the author supports the general consensus that treatment for stable portwine stain should be withheld until after puberty."[7] An early misconception was that treatment was not carried out in children because it was extremely difficult, if not impossible, under local anesthetic.[8] Even when general anesthetic facilities have been available it has still not been possible to obtain consistently good results in children; relatively few papers claim regularly to obtain good results in this age group. An exception is the paper by Brauner et al., who stress the importance of postoperative skin care in the reduction of scarring.[4] The argon laser treatment of children is discussed in more detail later in this chapter.

Using the noninvasive technique of transcutaneous microscopy, first described in this field by Shakespeare and Carruth,[9] it appears that a port-wine stain in young patients is commonly composed of a large number of relatively normal capillaries in which there does not seem to be an adequate "hemoglobin target" as defined by Noe et al.[10] There also appears to be a general consensus that the Argon laser produces better results in the treatment of facial lesions than of those on the limbs or trunk. This difference is certainly related to the technical problem of erasing a large mark on the body with a free-hand technique using a spot size of only 1.0 mm diameter.

Techniques Available To Aid Prediction of a Successful Outcome

Histology

Noe et al.[10] have shown that certain histologic features of a port-wine stain can be of value in the prediction of a good response. They studied the volume of the dermis occupied by vessels, the mean area of the cross section of the vessels, and the degree of filling of these vessels with erythrocytes. They showed that high values indicated a likely good result and referred to the "hemoglobin target" mentioned above each birthmark. Similarly, Ohmori and Huang[11] divided port-wine stains into four groups: constricted, intermediate, dilated, and deeply located. The constricted type of blood vessels differed very little from the normal pattern and number. In the dilated type the vessels were considerably enlarged (up to 400 μm) with a high content of red cells, and in the deep type the vessels were found scattered throughout the upper and lower dermis. The intermediate type showed histologic features common to the other forms mentioned.

Although a biopsy is, perhaps, the optimal method of prediction, and also of the assessment of results, it is an invasive technique that may not be acceptable to all patients, particularly those with a facial lesion. Certainly, regular followup by repeated biopsies is almost invariably not possible.

This lack of histologic followup is an additional reason why progress in the Argon-laser treatment of port-wine stains has been almost exclusively by the trial-and-error approach. With the widely used "minimal blanching technique," for example, the dermal depth of vascular injury seems never to have been assessed! Yet, it was recently shown by Tan et al.[12] that vascular injury deeper than 1 mm is required to fully erase a port-wine stain (this study was performed with the pulsed dye laser).

Noninvasive Techniques

Spectrophotometry. In the assessment of a patient Ohmori and Huang[11] showed that, using a spectrophotometer, there was an excellent correlation between the color of the birthmark and its histologic pattern as they had defined it. This instrument has been used both in the prediction of a successful outcome and in the objective followup assessment of patients; but, as mentioned earlier, spectrophotometrically excellent results do not always correlate with the clinical picture.

Transcutaneous Microscopy. This technique[9] enables the vessels comprising the port-wine stain to be examined through the intact epidermis following a simple application of liquid paraffin. Six different types of birthmark have been identified that correlate well with the histologic types described above. The technique has great potential for the assessment of patients before treatment and, indeed, at all stages of the treatment program. An unequivocal description of the PWS response to treatment is provided and, in addition to clearance of vessels, recognition of the abnormal vessels related to hypertrophic scarring is possible. The final role of transcutaneous microscopy in the prediction of the response of the PWS birthmark to any form of laser treatment remains to be defined, but there is already evidence[13] that the technique may be of value in assisting the prediction of a successful outcome.

Other Techniques. These include the use of various "flow meters" to assess the vascular dynamics of a birthmark as described by Apfelberg et al.[14] A noninvasive technique, however, has yet to be found to enable an accurate prediction of the outcome of laser treatment.

Test Patch

In view of the inability to predict accurately a successful outcome, a majority of workers carry out a test patch. In addition to the help this provides in predicting the response, it also enables the patient to see the changes that will occur in the treated area. The test patch may, on occasion, deter a patient from continuing with treatment. However, some workers who have developed a standardized technique, and in particular those who use a robotized, computerized hand piece or scanning device, debate whether a test patch is still necessary.

The range of treatment techniques will be discussed in detail in the following section. It is sufficient here to state that whatever treatment is employed by the individual practitioner, the same technique will be used for both the test patch and the subsequent treatment. Usually under a local anesthetic the laser is used to erase a thumbnail-sized test area. It is common practice to carry out a test on an inconspicuous area of the face, avoiding those areas which are notorious for scarring. The test is usually carried out at the junction of normal skin to birthmark, enabling easy comparison with both the untreated lesion and the normal skin. As is usual with the argon laser, the test area weeps serum for 1 to 2 days, or it may form a blister, followed by light crusting for up to 1 week. When the crusting separates, the tested area is still red. The color gradually fades until the test patch is judged after 6 months.

In the assessment of a test there are three possible results. First, a good/excellent result in which the color of the lesion has been satisfactorily reduced with preservation of normal skin texture; in these cases treatment will be carried out using the identical parameters. Second, the lesion is still too colored; in these cases many workers carry out a second test patch using higher power levels. In the author's experience, having used "minimal blanching power" for the first test, a second test is necessary in approximately 20% of patients [Carruth, unpublished results]; the power is increased by 0.2 W (typically in the range from 0.6 W to 1.5 W). The third possible result is that the patient may show atrophic or hypertrophic scarring in the tested area. If this occurs in a mature patient, then treatment will probably not be possible if minimal blanching power was used for the first test; but if it occurs in the younger patient, then it may be appropriate to carry out a further test at a later date.

Treatment Techniques

A vast range of treatment techniques has been described in the literature, but, as mentioned above, none of the techniques approaches the "ideal" as described by van Gemert et al. in Chapter 2 of this book. In all the techniques the irradiation time is several orders of magnitude greater than the theoretic ideal. This may explain why almost all the techniques give an approximately similar rate of good/excellent results and a similar rate of scarring.

Important parameters are the power, spot size, and irradiation time. These enable the power density (irradiance) and the incident-energy density of the beam to be calculated. With a free-hand technique these parameters are often difficult to measure. This is particularly so for the exposure time when a continuous expose technique is used; an "intermittent pulse technique," however, normally uses pulses of known duration.

Spot Size

The majority of hand pieces for the free-hand technique focus the beam from a distance of 2 to 4 cm on to the skin. No matter how careful the surgeon, there will be marked variations in the angle of the beam on the skin. This causes variations in the overall shape and size of the spot. Similarly, movement of the beam out of focus will change its size. The amounts by which the spot size will change was shown by Carruth,[6] but few workers use a spacer such as described in that paper to ensure a constant angle of the beam to the skin and precise focusing of the spot. As an example, a laser power of 1 W with a 1 mm diameter spot produces a power density of 127 W/cm^2. However, if the beam is defocused, either by moving it in or out from the focal point or by angling the beam to produce a spot size of, e.g., 1.2 mm diameter, the power density falls to 71.5 W/cm^2. It is therefore vital to ensure, either by careful technique or by some mechanical means, that the beam is kept both at a right angle to the skin and at the focal distance from it.

The majority of workers use a spot size of 1 mm diameter, although spot sizes as small as 0.1 mm diameter and as large as 5 mm diameter have been described in the literature.

The size of the spot will obviously affect the speed with which treatment can be carried out, and it will also have a significant effect on the depth of light penetration and, hence, on the final clinical result. This is owing to the influence of scattering. To illustrate this, Figure 2–3 in the earlier chapter by van Gemert et al. shows fluence rate distributions as a function of laser beam size. At an equal incident power density, small beams penetrate less deeply than large beams.

Consider now a PWS treatment with a very small spot size of 0.1 mm diameter. Such an example was investigated by Orenstein and Nelson[15] using the continuous wave (CW) 577 nm dye laser at 0.7 to 1 W/cm^2, with an irradiation time of 0.05 or 0.1 s, resulting in power densities of 900 to 12,000 W/cm^2 and incident-energy densities of 450 to 1200 joules/cm^2. Compare this to the Candela pulsed dye laser with 5 mm spot size, 0.45 ms irradiation time, an incident-energy density of 7 joules/cm^2, and a power density of 16,000 W/cm^2 (which is 1.3 to 1.7 times larger than that of the CW dye laser). On the (reasonable) assumption that the vascular damage mechanisms are similar for both systems, the pulsed dye laser has two substantial advantages over the continuous-wave small spot laser. First, even for identical power densities, a 5 mm laser spot has substantially deeper tissue penetration than a 0.1 mm spot. Second, deeper vascular coagulation depths are achieved with the pulsed dye laser at 64 to 186 times lower incident-energy densities. Additionally, a large spot, and hence deep light penetration, with very selective absorption by blood confines the light energy to the target blood vessels. It is a misconception that with small spot sizes "the energy would theoretically be more confined to the vessels as opposed to a larger spot." However, the large radial heat conduction that occurs when extremely small spot sizes are applied might explain why higher-power densities generated in small spots enable "the incident radiation to penetrate through the epidermis."[15]

Power

Using a 1 mm spot, Bard Cosman developed a technique described in a series of papers in 1980[16] and 1982[17] in which he employed for the first time "minimal power argon laser therapy." This technique has been developed and slightly renamed by one of the authors (JASC) as the "minimal blanching power technique." To determine the required power for this technique, the beam, using either intermittent pulsed or continuous exposure, is moved across the birthmark while the power is raised from 0.4 W, in increments of 0.2 W, until at a particular power (usually between 0.6 and 1.2 W) minimal blanching occurs. Subsequently, this power is used to carry out both the test and, if the test is successful, the treatment.

If a particular power density has been selected, it is not possible with the majority of clinical lasers to use much larger spot sizes because the laser is unable to produce sufficient total power. (As the area of the spot depends on the square of the radius, doubling the radius means increasing the power by a factor of four to produce the same power density.) Some workers, however, do use much higher power levels, on the order of 5 or even 6 W on a 1 mm spot, but claim to produce the same total energy density by moving the beam rapidly over the tissue.[18] Other workers, like Hulsbergen-Henning,[19] use a 2 mm spot size, high power levels up to 10 W, and short irradiation times of 0.05 s or less.

Exposure Time

Much of the early work was carried out with an intermittent exposure of 0.2 s. Intermittent pulse techniques are still used by some workers and form the basis of the Hexascan computerized hand piece. However, for free-hand work with a small spot and intermittent pulse technique, this was found to be extremely tedious and time consuming, and the majority of workers now use a continuous beam "air brush technique."

Arndt [1984] clinically compared short (0.05 s) with longer irradiation conditions in a total of 27 patients. Unfortunately, because the incident-energy density was not kept constant, his conclusion that there was no significant difference in blanching must be interpreted with caution. Recently, J.P. Hulsbergen-Henning stated, on the basis of clinical evidence, that short irradiation times (< 0.05 s) produce better clinical results than longer times, especially less hypopigmentation and less atrophy; the incidence of hypertrophic scarring is expected to be reduced as well.[19] Similarly, Pickering et al. found a clinical improvement with copper vapor laser treatment at shorter (0.03 s) compared with longer (0.1 s) irradiation times.[20]

Energy Density

The total energy density (joules/cm^2) is calculated by multiplying the power density with the exposure time. The same energy density may be achieved by using a low-power density with long exposure or a high-power density with short exposure. At the two extremes of these techniques are that of the author, who uses low power and a slow speed of the continuous beam across the tissue monitored by the achievement of clinical blanching, and that described by the workers in Toulouse,[18] where a much higher power density is used and the beam is moved rapidly and systematically over the lesion. As mentioned above, it is obviously possible to measure exactly the treatment energy if an intermittent pulse of 0.2 s is used; but with continuous exposure and an "air-brush" technique it is difficult, if not impossible, to measure the total energy. However, with the new computerized scanners, which move the beam automatically at constant speed over the tissues, this problem has been overcome.

Erasure Techniques

With a hand-held technique several different erasure methods have been adopted. The first uses a "spot by spot" technique. Among workers with this method debate has always existed whether the spots should be immediately adjacent to each other or should overlap to give a more uniform clinical erasure but with, perhaps, a greater chance of scarring. With the author's early spotting technique, using overlapping spots,[21] it was found that the treated area as measured by the spot size and number of impacts was 1.5 times the measured treated area on the skin. Apfelberg et al.[22] have introduced a pointillistic technique in which treated spots are separated by a distance of 1.0 to 2.0 mm, and the unblanched areas are treated at a later date. With this he suggests that a lower rate of scarring may be achieved, and there should be no unsightly evidence of the spotting found to be a problem with his earlier striped techniques.

When the beam is used in a continuous mode, it is moved along the natural lines of the skin to erase the mark, using minimal blanching as the end point. As previously mentioned, the speed of movement depends on the power density of the beam. Naturally, it is more difficult and requires more skill to move the beam at high speed with precision and at a regular pace.

Apfelberg[23] introduced his zebra stripe technique in which treated stripes were separated by untreated ones; from this procedure it was thought that better epidermal regeneration could occur. In a subsequent paper,[24] however, he stated that the technique had been abandoned, as there was almost invariably residual striping of the treated mark that adversely affected the final cosmetic result.

Whichever technique is employed undoubtedly demands a high degree of expertise to produce consistently satisfactory results, and these results have a poor reproducibility in other hands and in other centers. It is essential to use a technique that can be employed on a wide range of birthmarks over an acceptable time span; clearly, the intermittent spot and the point techniques are slow and time consuming. If a continuous beam technique is used with contiguous or overlapping lines along the natural skin lines of the face, then better and more consistent erasure can be obtained in a much shorter period of time. Although it may seem reasonable to expect that this technique will produce a greater chance of scar formation, such has not regularly been shown in the literature.

Each technique has its advantages and its drawbacks, but all appear to share the limitations of poor reproducibility, lack of homogeneous energy delivery, and a relative inability to treat large birthmarks. It would appear that the only way to overcome these limitations consistently with a high degree of reproducibility is by the introduction of computerized systems of treatment.

Automated Treatment Devices

Many workers have made attempts to devise and develop automated treatment systems. With the present sophistication of robots it should be possible to produce a system to treat all birthmarks in a totally automatic fashion. Unfortunately, such a system would most likely be too expensive for widespread clinical usage. However, four systems that appear to offer particular promise in this field have recently been introduced. Delacrétaz et al.[25] have described a scanning system composed of two mirrors independently driven by galvanometric scanners. The spot is automatically scanned with constant laser power over the desired area; the velocity of scanning is adjusted to obtain an appropriate incident irradiance. The Telescan developed by Laffitte et al.[18] appears to be a similar system; some encouraging preliminary results have been reported.

In New Zealand, a computer-controlled, mirror-based scanner has been developed by Walker and his team[26] for use with the copper vapor laser,[26a] which, they believe, has significant advantages over the argon laser. With this scanner the spot can be moved at a totally controllable speed over the lesion, enabling precise but rather linear erasure to be performed. Another promising system is the hexascan described by Mordon et al.[27] This comprises a microprocessor-controlled hand piece allowing precise measurement and delivery of laser energy. A hexagonal mask placed on the area to be treated is filled in automatically by a spotting technique, so designed to ensure that there is an appropriate time for cooling between the delivery of adjacent spots. Irradiation time per spot is variable from 0.03 s and longer. Because of the precise control of the spots a high degree of homogeneity of blanching can be achieved. In addition, it is stated that the treatment time is reduced by approximately 20% compared to the conventional, manual point-by-point method. A wide range of port-wine stains and other vascular lesions has been treated with this scanner; results appear to be reproducible and superior to those achieved by a hand-held technique.

Anesthesia

Certain centers maintain that argon laser therapy can be carried out without any form of anesthesia in adults, particularly when a point-by-point technique is used; but in the experience of the author few patients in Britain would tolerate this. EMLA cream may be used to reduce—but it does not totally abolish—the pain of treatment. Much of the work with the argon laser is carried out under local anesthetic given by injection. The choice of local anesthetic will depend on the individual practitioner, but it should not contain epinephrine, as this may effect the blood vessels, and it should be given deeply under the lesion to avoid hydrostatic distortion of the vessels. If children are to be treated, a general anesthetic will often be needed. Similarly, this may also be needed for the treatment of nervous adults.

Results

As detailed above it is difficult, if not impossible, to make accurate comments on the results from the various series described in the literature. A review of the results by Touquet and Carruth[21] and by Silver [28] shows that excellent/good results occurred in 60 to 75% of cases and scarring in 5 to 20%. However, in the series reported by Masser et al.,[13] when any textural change in the skin was regarded as scarring, the incidence approached 50%.

Gilchrest et al., in a study of 30 patients,[29] reported that it was possible to improve the results by chilling the skin before treatment. These observations were confirmed later by Dréno et al. in 40 patients,[30] but Yanai et al. found no clinical improvement in 101 patients.[31] Therefore, it seems uncertain whether chilling the skin before treatment will improve the clinical outcome. The authors who observed a positive effect were unable to give a clear explanation.

Cosman[17] showed with minimal-power argon laser treatment that retreatment could be performed after 15 to 18 months with further cosmetic improvement and with a chance of scarring no higher than that of the original treatment.

Treatment of Children

The treatment of PWS birthmarks in children is of particular interest, as all would wish to relieve the patient of the stigma of the port-wine stain at the earliest possible moment. Yet the argon laser treatment of children remains controversial. There appears to be a general consensus that treatment should not be carried out until after puberty in view of the poor prognosis for a successful result and also from the standpoint of an increased risk of hypertrophic scarring.[32] However, these views are not fully supported by a study of the literature.

In 13 patients, Dixon et al.[3] found that the incidence of hypertrophic scarring in children under of 12 years of age may approach 40%. It would appear from a number of series,[4,13] however, that children are still being treated, and Lannigan and Cotterill[33] report successful results in the treatment of pale lesions in children using the carbon dioxide laser.

In 1978 Ohmori et al.[34] reported a series of 437 patients of whom 311 were below 16 years of age. These authors reported 6.6% excellent results (total blanching without scar), 69.1% good (marked lightening without scar), and 24.3% fair (limited improvement). Keloid formation occurred in 2.2% and uneven scars in 5.5% of the cases. Unfortunately, the results and side effects were not separated into children and adults. But if one assumes that *all* the hypertrophic scarring were produced in children, this would result in only 3.2% of keloids and 8% of uneven scars with a total incidence of 11.2% of scarring. Brauner et al.[4] published a large series of 84 children younger than 13 years of age with a followup period of at least 6 months. Their overall results were: 7% excellent (total clearing), 53% good (moderate to marked clearing), 21% fair, and 15% poor. The incidence of hypertrophic scarring was 8%; however, the authors remark that these 7 patients were treated (by the late Dr. Bard Cosman) in the early quarter of the study with much higher energy fluences of 22 to 38 J/cm^2, compared with 10 to 15 J/cm^2 in the later part of the series. In addition, in the early part of the series no careful postoperative wound care was carried out, and the authors claim that children can be successfully treated in approximately 60% of cases with a minimal blanching technique using a 1.5 mm spot and a pulse duration of 0.2 seconds. They consider that hypertrophic scarring should not occur if careful post-treatment wound care is carried out: that is, immediate chilling for 2 or more minutes with an ice pack, and the application of antibacterial ointment and an occlusive dressing. The semipermeable dressing and the antibiotic cream should be changed daily. These results are in contrast with those reported by Masser et al.,[13] who treated 11 children under the age of 13 years in essentially an identical fashion but did not use any form of dressing in the postoperative period; they reported an incidence of scarring of more than 50% (although, as mentioned earlier, any change in skin texture was reported as scarring). In addition, Noe[32] reported in 12 patients younger than 17 years of age an incidence of 25% of hypertrophic scarring (3 patients) and 4 additional patients who showed insufficient blanching.

In the authors' experience,[35] and referring to Masser's paper, more than 50 children have been treated with only 2 excellent results, and in 11 other patients treatment was abandoned owing to a poor outcome. The remaining subjects are still under evaluation, but no new patients under the age of 20 are now being treated in Southampton with the argon laser.

The problem of hypertrophic scarring is especially vexatious since no truly satisfactory definition of a hypertrophic scar exists. Such scars occur frequently after burn injuries in children, and approximately 50% of those treated at the Wessex Regional Burns Unit require followup for hypertrophic scarring.[36] The treatment may deal with only a very minor problem or with an extensive development of scars, so these figures represent only a crude indication of the outcome of healing. It is not known whether the incidence of hypertrophic scarring in children after burn injury is higher than that among adults. The different causes of burn injuries in children (85% scald injury) compared with adults (20% scald, 40% flame burns) complicates the issue. There is also the probability that higher concern for minor hypertrophic scarring in children influences the apparent incidence of the condition. It is therefore difficult to assess with confidence that children are "more prone" to hypertrophic scarring than adults.

Possibly the difficulties in treating children arise from the nature of the port-wine stain in children rather than from any innate predisposition to scarring. In the 40 children under treatment in Southampton who have been investigated by transcutaneous microscopy, a majority of the lesions has been classified as type A or B lesions, which contain relatively normal vessels. These vessels (with very short relaxation times) transmit a greater proportion of the heat generated to the surrounding tissue matrix than do larger vessels of mature lesions. The proportion of such "minimal structural deviation" lesions that occurs in adults is very much lower.[35]

The controversy with regard to the treatment of children remains unsolved, and the "consensus" that satisfactory results cannot always be obtained in children may relate to the structure of the birthmark rather than to the age of the patient. It must be pointed out, however, that if a minimal blanching power technique is used in children, and one assumes that the optical absorption and scattering properties of the skin are similar in children and adults, then a deeper thermal damage will be produced in children relative to the overall thickness of the skin compared with adults. In addition to this, Cosman[16] reported that, especially in areas that are at risk for hypertrophic scarring, such as on the upper lip, the argon laser power required for minimal blanching "dropped by one-half as the nasolabial fold was crossed from cheek to lip."

In conclusion, these results suggest, especially in the treatment of children, that clinical experience, in addition to an extremely careful choice of laser parameters and adequate postoperative wound care, plays a vitally important role in the prevention of hypertrophic scarring.

Conclusions

Is it possible to draw significant conclusions on the role of the Argon laser? The answer must be yes, and it certainly does provide "a ray of hope" for the successful treatment of many patients.[37] The ultimate aim of laser therapy for port-wine stain birthmarks must be to treat patients at the earliest possible age to avoid the immense psychologic damage a PWS birthmark may cause. Unfortunately, with the Argon laser, this aim has not been realized in a majority of the published literature. Some recent papers do offer hope for young patients treated with this laser using a minimal-power technique and careful postoperative wound care. But careful comparison with the pulsed dye laser is required before the role of the argon laser in the treatment of children can be finally assessed.

For the treatment of the mature birthmark the introduction of scanning systems will undoubtedly improve the quality of the results and their reproducibility. This will require a substantial financial outlay, approximately one-half the cost of an argon laser. It would appear certain, however, that automated techniques will totally replace the free-hand techniques in the near future.

The problem remains that argon lasers are not available that will produce the "ideal treatment parameters" (high power and millisecond irradiation time) for laser therapy of port-wine stains. If machines producing these parameters were widely available, then it would be possible to re-evaluate the argon laser and to make precise comparisons of the results achieved by this laser with those achieved using the pulsed dye laser, whose parameters more closely approach the "ideal."

Finally, from the results obtained with the pulsed dye laser, one has every reason to believe that the "theoretically ideal parameters" are accurate, and on that basis to say that the argon laser has never truly been used in an optimal fashion. Considering this fact, the results achieved with this laser are remarkably good, and with further development in the parameters and in the use of automated treatment devices the results must surely improve in the next decade.

References

1. Apfelberg DB, Kosek J, Maser MR, Lash H. Histology of portwine stains following argon laser treatment. Br J Plast Surg 32:232, 1979.
2. Finley JL, Brasky SH, Geer DE, et al. Healing of port wine stains after argon laser therapy. Arch Dermatol 117:486, 1981.
3. Dixon JA, Huether S, Rotering R. Hypertrophic scarring in argon laser treatment of port-wine stains. Plast Reconstr Surg 73:771, 1984.
4. Brauner G, Schilftman A, Cosman B. Evaluation of Argon laser surgery in children under 13 years of age. Plast Reconstr Surg 87:37, 1991.

5. Quaba AA. Results of argon laser treatment of portwine stains: a method of assessment. Br J Plast Surg 42:125, 1989.

6. Carruth JAS. The establishment of precise physical parameters for the treatment of the portwine stain with the argon laser. Lasers Surg Med 2:37, 1982.

7. Hobby LW. Argon laser treatment of superficial vascular lesion in children. Lasers Surg Med 6:16, 1986.

8. Carruth JAS. Lasers in dermatology. *In* New Clinical Applications in Dermatology and Surgery. Edited by J Verbov. Lancaster (England), MTP Press, pp 27–77, 1986, p 27.

9. Shakespeare PG, Carruth JAS. Investigating the structure of the portwine stain by transcutaneous microscopy. Lasers Med Sci 1:107, 1986.

10. Noe JM, Barsky SH, Geer DE, Rosen S. Portwine stains and the response to argon laser therapy: successful treatment and the predictive role of color, age and biopsy. Plast Reconstr Surg 65:130, 1980.

10a. Arndt KA. Treatment techniques in argon laser therapy: Comparison of pulse and continuous exposures. J Am Acad Dermatol 11:90, 1984.

11. Ohmori S, Huan CK. Recent progress in the treatment of port wine staining by the argon laser: some observations on the prognostic value of relative spectroreflectance (R.S.R.) and the histological classification of the lesions. Br J Plast Surg 34:249, 1981.

12. Tan OT, Morisson P, Kurban AK. 585 nm for the treatment of port-wine stains. Plast Reconstr Surg 86:1112, 1990.

13. Masser MR, Sammut DP, Jones SG, Saxby PJ. Argon laser therapy of port-wine stains—prediction of the effect by transcutaneous microscopy. Lasers Med Sci 4:237, 1989.

14. Apfelberg DB, Smith T, White J. Preliminary study of the vascular dynamics of the portwine hemangioma with therapeutic implications of argon laser treatment. Plast Reconstr Surg 83:820, 1989.

15. Orenstein A, Nelson JS. Treatment of facial vascular lesions with a 100-micrometer spot 577-nm pulsed continuous wave dye laser. Ann Plast Surg 23:310, 1989.

16. Cosman B. Clinical experience in the laser therapy of port wine stains. Lasers Surg Med 1:133, 1980.

17. Cosman B. Role of retreatment in minimal power argon laser therapy for portwine stains. Lasers Surg Med 2:43, 1982.

18. Laffitte F, Chavoin JP, Rouge D, Costagliola M. Automatic scanning for argon laser treatment of large PWS. Abstract from 4th Biennial Meeting of the European Laser Association. Lasers Med Sci 3:235, 1988.

19. Hulsbergen-Henning JP (Veldhoven, The Netherlands) in a private communication to van Gemert. To be published.

20. Pickering JW, Walker EP, Butler PH, Halewijn CN van. Copper vapour laser treatment of port-wine stains and other vascular malformations. Br J Plast Surg 43:273, 1990.

21. Touquet VLR, Carruth JAS. Review of the treatment of portwine stains with the argon laser. Lasers Surg Med 4:191, 1984.

22. Apfelberg DB, Smith T, Maser MR, et al. Dot or pointillistic method for improvement in results of hyperactive scarring in the argon laser treatment of portwine hemangioma. Lasers Surg Med 6:558, 1987.

23. Apfelberg DB, Maser MR, Lash H, Rivers JL. Progress report on extended clinical use of the argon laser for cutaneous lesions. Lasers Surg Med 1:70, 1980.

24. Apfelberg DB, Flores JT, Maser MR, Lash H. Analysis of complications of argon laser treatment for portwine stain haemangioma with reference to the stripe technique. Lasers Surg Med 2:357, 1983.

25. Delacrétaz G, Polla LL, Wöste L. Scanning CW dye (577 nm) laser device for selective vessel photothermolysis. Proc 9th Annu Meet Am Soc Laser Med Surg 176:43 (abstract), 1989.

26. Smithies DJ, Butler PH, Pickering JW, Walker EP. A computer controlled scanner for the laser treatment of vascular lesions and hyperpigmentation. Clin Phys Physiol Meas 1991 (in press).

26a. Walker EP, Butler PH, Pickering JW. Histology of portwine stains of the copper vapour laser treatment. Br J Dermatol 121:217, 1989.

27. Mordon S, Rotteleur G, Buys B, Brunetaud JM. Comparative study of the ''point-by-point technique'' and the ''scanning technique'' for laser treatment of port-wine stains. Lasers Surg Med 4:398, 1989.

28. Silver L. Argon laser photocoagulation of the portwine stain haemangiomas. Lasers Surg Med 6:20, 1986.

29. Gilchrest BA, Rosen S, Noe JM. Chilling portwine stains improves the response to argon laser treatment. Plast Reconstr Surg 69:278, 1982.

30. Dréno B, Patrice T, Litoux P, Barrière H. The benefit of chilling in argon-laser treatment of port-wine stains. Plast Reconstr Surg 75:42, 1985.

31. Yanai A, Fukuda O, Soyano S, et al. Argon laser therapy of port-wine stains: effects and limitations. Plast Reconstr Surg 75:520, 1985.

32. Noe JM. Discussion on hypertrophic scarring in argon laser treatment of portwine stains. Plast Reconstr Surg 73:778, 1984.
33. Lannigan SW, Cotterill JA. The treatment of portwine stains with the CO_2 laser. Br J Dermatol 123:229, 1990.
34. Ohmori S, Huang CK, Takada H, et al. Experience with the treatment of portwine stain with argon laser beam. *In* Laser Surgery II. Edited by I Kaplan. Jerusalem, Jerusalem Academic Press, 1978, p 256.
35. Carruth JAS, Shakespeare PG. Unpublished results.
36. Spurr ED, Shakespeare PG. Incidence of hypertrophic scarring in burn-injured children. Burns, 16:179, 1990.
37. Editorial. New ray of hope for portwine stains. Lancet 1:480, 1981.

Additional Readings

Carruth JAS, Shakespeare PG. Towards the ideal treatment for the portwine stain with the argon laser: better prediction and an 'optimal' technique. Lasers Surg Med 6:2, 1986.
Gemert MJC van, Welch AJ, Amin AP. Is there an optimal laser treatment for portwine stains? Lasers Surg Med 6:76, 1986.
Gemert MJC van, Welch AJ, Miller ID, Tan OT. Can physical modeling lead to an optimal laser treatment strategy for port-wine stains? *In* ML Wolbarsht. Laser applications in medicine and biology. Edited by ML Wolbarsht. New York, Plenum Press, 1991, p 199.
Larrow L, Noe JM. Portwine stain haemangioma. Am J Nurs 82:786, 1982.

Chapter 5   The Role of Anesthesia in Laser Therapy

Timothy J. Stafford
Dean Crocker

The potential for pain exists in all surgery, including minor dermatologic laser surgery. To the extent that this pain is traumatic to the patient or limits or inhibits the surgery it becomes a major component of the total operational experience. In this very brief review we attempt to describe the laser-induced pain in the context of its currently known mechanisms; we refer specifically to children, who are a particularly large group of the patients.

In reviewing the potential methods of pain control in this type of surgery, we place particular emphasis on general anesthesia, its practical requirements, and its potential complications, since in many centers this is a method commonly employed.

As well as other centrally directed techniques of analgesia, including systemic analgesics and sedatives, other methods include the use of local anesthetics, with a wide range of routes of administration, systemic, regional, topical. Although these drugs are relatively safe, they also involve complications, and an understanding of their pharmacology is essential even in the least invasive application.

The new development in topical anesthesia, based on the lidocaine-prilocaine combination of local anesthetics, EMLA, seems to be so noninvasive that, in a range of analgesic techniques, it perhaps can represent the other end of the spectrum from general anesthesia. In the final choice of technique, the clinician balances risk and benefit.

The Pain of Laser Surgery

The characteristics and degree of pain associated with the pulsed dye laser treatment of skin have been well described. Initially there is a "sharp stinging pain," which has been likened to the snap of a rubber band against the skin. With this there is a sensation of mechanical impact, distinct from, for example, a pin prick, that indeed has been postulated to relate to a localized shock wave. Accompanying this "skin shock" is a second distinct heat sensation, which can be at least as unpleasant as the initial sting. While it also rapidly fades, it seems to build up if successive pulses are closely approximated over a confined area over a short time, as is the normal technique of treating a port-wine stain (PWS) birthmark. This increasing pain to subsequent laser pulses is noted over both the immediate area of the injury and also the surrounding area.

In general there seems to be little difference in sensation over PWS skin and normal skin. Subsequently over a few minutes, an itch develops which lasts a variable period, and in most individuals it subsides in half an hour or so.

Campbell[1] classifies the nociceptive fiber types in skin as slow-conducting unmyelinated C-fibers polymodally responsive to mechanical and heat stimuli (CMH), responsible for the second burning pain of a heat trauma; and myelinated A-fibers (AMH), divided into type I, responsible for the primary hyperalgesia, and type II, the fastest-conducting type, associated with the first pricking pain.

It can also be postulated that the mechanical shock sensation accompanying the first pricking pain as the laser energy is dissipated might also be attributable to the stimulus of a distinct group of high-threshold, purely mechanically responsive receptors.

The sensation of itch is less clear-cut. There do not appear to be distinct fibers associated with this sensation that may be due to central processing.

Such a description is consistently reported by adults who can discriminate sensation based on the experience of pain and can verbalize it. In degree, most such observers liken the discomfort to the vertical penetration of the superficial skin by a fine 25-gauge needle. However, there are wide variations. Not surprisingly, anatomic location is important. Certain areas of the face and the digits particularly are very dense in nerve endings, and trauma in these locations produces more pain. It is unfortunate that the location of PWS in patients presenting for treatment tends, statistically, to be precisely in these areas — the exposed surfaces of the normally clothed individual.[2] Then again, over and above this, the digits often present specific pain problems. In some patients, PWS involving the digits is associated with a deeper vascular-pathologic condition producing engorged and tense tissue that seems to be particularly sensitive to the laser.

Other dimensions of variability have been reported. Diurnal variation has been cited,[3] but unfortunately with distinct results from study to study. Regarding gender, there appears to be no difference between the sexes in pain *threshold;* adult males, however, appear to demonstrate more *tolerance* of pain than females.[4] By discriminating tolerance from threshold we have expanded the construct of pain from the purely physiologic to the much wider dimension of pain as subjective and responsive. In the clinical setting this dimension is much more relevant, particularly when we are considering skin laser treatment that produces short, sharp pain in awake patients, and particularly when a large proportion of these patients is children.

Children and the Pain Response

All clinicians are familiar with the wide variation in tolerance with which children will respond to a standardized trauma, an immunization shot, or an intravenous placement (levels of stimulation, incidentally, which are probably not dissimilar to the laser impact). Certainly a basic predisposition exists in an individual in his reactivity to the pain stimulus, and this seems to be a learned phenomenon. The experienced observer will further note that, although certain children can be more tolerant than others, their state is at all times potentially subject to the occasion, the environment, and a host of other factors. The particular interaction on a specific occasion with accompanying family or clinical staff will be significant.[5]

Parents can be overreactive, perhaps deriving secondary gain from the stance of the ''caring'' protector or from their own anxiety; they can be oversolicitous to their child's pain events, thereby rewarding the child for inappropriate responses. Children's behavioral responses to pain can be acquired from the parents, the family, and peers. The peer response can be particularly important as children get older. Likewise, film and video models have been described as very effective in creating new behaviors and response patterns among growing children.

In the context of the PWS laser treatment, an important factor is the short-period, repetitive nature of the pain stimulus. Anticipation of the pain experience clearly is a major factor in the response behavior. Mittwoch et al.,[6] using electric shock as the pain event, have examined aversiveness to pain in relation to both instructed pain-coping techniques and the warning period before the pain event. They found that the pain-coping instruction they employed had no significance, whereas a short warning period, 5 seconds, produced less ''pain rating'' and anxiety than longer periods. (This 5-second period, interestingly, closely approximates the pulse-to-pulse recharging interval which treatment of a skin surface by the pulsed dye laser requires.) Despite this study, Ross and Ross[5] place great emphasis on the modification to pain behavior that can result from control methods taught to children.

Hypnosis and the Pain Response in Children

The concept of hypnosis in the management of acute pain is, to many clinicians, something both esoteric and alarming. Many physicians in particular, trained in the context of specific interventions with a powerful pharmacopeia, feel uncomfortable with the idea. Yet there is overwhelming evidence that the psychologic status of the patient has a powerful influence on the perception of pain, both acute and chronic; and we also have a strong theoretic construct of descending pathways of modulation to peripheral pain stimuli.

A useful way to view hypnosis is not as a technique of control by the hypnotist, but as a subject's method of self-control. The hypnotist ''coaches'' the subject to relax, modify his own state of consciousness, and, in this context, modulate the response to the noxious stimulus.

Clinicians who are very experienced with children informally develop ways of enabling the child to respond well to a painful event. The successful practitioners often concentrate on engaging the child to perform some simple maneuver such as steady breathing. Such interactions can often be seen as paralleling formal hypnosis. We find that timing the pain event, be it pin prick or laser shot, to expiration can be less traumatic. The key factor is to include the child in the process, giving him some degree of control, some mechanism of coping. Ross and Ross detail a wide range of processes by which children faced with recurrent painful stimuli (burns' dressing changes, e.g.) themselves create methods of coping.

The role of the clinician is to help and coach the child. This is distinct from distracting the child. Extreme distractions, such as cartoons, can be useful but can indeed be counterproductive.

Methods of Pain Control

In response to pain arising in the context of therapeutic procedural intervention, physicians employ pharmacologic pain control in three categories: full general anesthesia; centrally acting drugs representing a lesser degree of central depression of cortical areas; and local anesthesia. Included in this last category are peripheral and central nerve blocks, field blocks, and topical anesthesia. Let us begin at one end of the spectrum, i.e., general anesthesia.

General Anesthesia

General anesthesia for pain control in laser surgery as in any surgery involves a number of requirements. In the majority of the United States the practice of anesthesia is held to a standard of care appropriate to the general community, that is, equal service, space, monitoring, and in general a modern protocol.

The first requirement to be addressed is a proper environment. Criteria of a designated anesthetizing location include the following:

1. Fixed number of square feet as designated by federal and state standards.
2. Isolation line transformers for prevention of leakage current to the electrical-sensitive patient.
3. Anesthesia machine with appropriate vaporizers and a program of biomedical testing to ensure accurate delivery of gas and vapor with "fail-safe" mechanisms acceptable to government standards.
4. Scavenging systems for waste gas to protect personnel, and a recordkeeping system of monitoring environment as prescribed by OSHA.
5. Monitoring systems including temperature with alarms for blood pressure, pulse, EKG, and respiratory parameters. It has became mandatory for malpractice coverage in some states to have "end tidal" carbon dioxide measurements and continuous oxygen-saturation measurement.
6. Resuscitation equipment including a pacemaker defibrillator, oxygen delivery system, intravenous drugs, and appropriately sized airway equipment.
7. Adequate personnel, including nursing, a safeguard in the event of an untoward reaction.
8. Recovery area equipment to standard with appropriately trained personnel.
9. Complete recordkeeping system by time.

General anesthesia is very resource-intensive and, owing to the necessity of conforming to various regulatory authorities, as well as for reasons of safety, is also very costly.

Once a proper environment for delivering general anesthesia for laser surgery has been established, the next criterion to be addressed is the work-up of the patient. History, especially of associated disease states such as diabetes, heart, and liver, must be elucidated and the appropriate laboratory tests performed before the choice of anesthetic agents can be decided. In the case of a child, a careful search for congenital anomalies should be carried out. The rule that single congenital anomalies rarely exist alone must be borne in mind; this is especially true in children with vascular malformations presenting for laser surgery. Associated arteriovenous fistulae such as occur in Sturge-Weber syndrome are not uncommon. One should listen to the child's head with a stethoscope in order to seek the "rush-like" hum. Arteriovenous malformations of the lung or abdomen may be present, and sometimes a history of bleeding tendencies will tip off the examiner to platelet trapping in these areas. Examination of the fontanelles in infants often will give clues to abnormal pulsations or increased intracranial pressure.

Blood volume of a small child should always be kept in mind. Although blood loss is rare, one would note that a loss of only 20 cc in a 5-pound infant (i.e., >10% loss) would require transfusion.

The essential point is that general anesthesia not only depresses physiologic functions such as cardiac contractility, but also suppresses protective autonomic controls. In children, the unforseen and anomalous may be accelerated under a general anesthesia.

As in any other form of therapy, one must address the risk/reward ratio. With general anesthesia, the risks are manifold, and one must justify the use of this modality. If there is no other method to accomplish the procedure, as in open heart surgery, the decision obviously must be general anesthesia. If there are alternatives, then relative risks must be examined.

One would ask, What are the risks? Allergic response, hypotension, nausea, vomiting, prolonged awakening, and a long list of minor responses are well known to any practioner, and are fairly common. Let us explore some of the more major complications. Major complications of general anesthesia (Table 5–1) relate primarily to the nervous system. They are usually related to a decrease in blood flow for even a brief period of time owing to

Table 5–1. Major Central Nervous System Complications of General Anesthesia

1. Emotional disturbances, temporary or permanent anxieties, personality changes
2. Behavior disturbances
3. Peripheral nerve palsies
4. Blindness
5. Spastic disorders, diplegia, quadriplegia
6. Seizure disorders
7. Mental retardation
8. Dementia
9. Decerebrate status
10. Death

Table 5–2. Death Rate for Children From General Anesthesia

Year	Total Cases	Deaths	Ratio of Deaths to Cases
1985	108,100	75	1:1,440
1986	117,800	80	1:1,470
1987	123,600	89	1:1,390
1988	122,000	72	1:1,690
1989	128,000	68	1:1,880

hypotension or cardiac arrest when there is insignificant oxygen transport to sensitive nerve cells.

With general anesthesia, prevention is much better than trying to correct a problem once it occurs. The recognized methods of prevention are:

1. The issue of proper "hospital" facilities
2. An experienced, trained, operating team
3. Proper preparation of the patient
4. Well-defined anesthesia management to include:

   - Correct drugs and dosages
   - Complete equipment
   - Monitoring
   - Patient observation
   - Back-up and support services

5. Appropriate postoperative care

The lessons of trying to cut corners or temporize have been learned by both physicians and patients over the years. The American Society of Anesthesia has developed a risk management oversight committee to develop standards for all aspects of general anesthesia; the committee studies the cases in which complications have occurred to develop policy and procedure.

The worst imaginable outcome of a general anesthesia is death. The commonly accepted estimates of death rate for adults range from 1/8,000 to 1/10,000. Because of malpractice considerations it is very difficult to obtain accurate current information. For children, the death rate is believed to be as shown in Table 5–2, which represents a survey of 6 major pediatric hospitals in the United States.

A survey of another 28 malpractice suits involving children yielded the following information:

1. Patient age: <1   1–6   6–12   12–20 years
   No. of patients   8   9   8   3

2. ASA Status: 1   1E   2   2E   3   3E   4   4E   5   5E
   No. of patients: 11   4   8   1   2   1   1   0   0   0

   Death   12
   Severe brain damage   13
   Neurologic defect   3

An analysis of these data shows the rather disconcerting fact that most anesthesia problems occurred in young healthy patients undergoing fairly minor procedures.

Centrally Acting Drugs

In addition to formal general anesthesia, there exists a much wider pharmacopeia that has been developed to work on different systems of the body in response to pain and other phenomena, both physiological and emotional. This would include hypnotics for sleep, opiates for pain, paralyzing agents for muscular relaxation, tranquilizers for fear, tricyclics and related drugs for depression, as well as many others such as "dissociative" agents that separate emotion from response. All these drugs have side effects that to varying degrees may produce discomfort or even life-threatening reactions in the patient.

An example is afforded by the drug ketamine, which is in common use. It was noted in *Science* that "there is an apparent neurotoxic effect of PCP and related agents (MK-801, tiletamine and ketamine), which has heretofore been overlooked: these drugs induce acute pathological changes in specific populations of brain nerves when administered subcutaneously to adult rats in low doses" (244:1360, 1989). In our litigious society this creates the possibility for the physician to be at malpractice risk for years—if little Johnny does not grow up as intelligent as Mommy and Daddy feel he has to be.

These general categories of opiates, hypnotics, and other centrally active drugs have a major drawback when used for definitive procedural therapy: that is, unpredictable specificity. The wide variety of factors in the individual's psyche, personality, response to stimulus and pain, fears, repressions, and general psychology makes it impossible to administer one or even a group of such drugs in a predictable fashion. They are useful in association with general anesthesia for relief of pain, or as mixed depressive pharmacologic agents.

When these centrally acting drugs are used in an attempt to mimic the "ideal" surgical conditions of general anesthesia in sedation and analgesia, then danger exists. As the adage states, "there are no minor anesthetics."

Local Anesthetic Techniques

For localization of the analgesic goal, an extremely wide range of techniques, difficult and complex, is available: thus spinal blocks, epidural blocks, regional intravenous blocks, major and minor nerve blocks, field blocks, infiltration blocks, and even topical blocks. All allow minimal interference and depression of the central nervous system. All are at least potentially applicable to and appropriate for dermatologic laser surgery. A good survey of the various methods is given in the *Handbook of Regional Anesthesia.*[7] What is central to all these methods is their reliance on a distinct class of drugs, the local anesthetics, a basic understanding of which should precede their use.

Local Anesthetics

The structurally similar compounds of this group produce reversible analgesia by intercepting electrical impulse conduction along nerves, and they act by blocking sodium channels in the nerve membrane, thereby inhibiting depolarization. While the target tissue for these drugs in their therapeutic role as analgesics is peripheral nerves, their pharmacologic action is on all excitable tissue; therefore, when side effects are considered, the central nervous system (CNS) and cardiac muscle are particularly important. CNS effects, manifest as drowsiness with epileptiform responses at high levels of toxicity, are well known, short-lived, and relatively manageable. Cardiac effects occur at higher doses.

In addition to the common toxicity problems, mention should be made of the methemoglobinemia associated with prilocaine.

Toxic levels for these drugs, which have different potencies, are shown in Table 5–3. The commonly used local anesthetics comprise two subgroups, the so-called amides and esters, classified according to the type of chemical linkage at one point of the molecule; this linkage is clinically important in hydrolytic stability and thereby offers a potential route of metabolism. Metabolism of the esters is effected by pseudocholinesterase, whereas the amides, stable to this enzyme, are hepatically metabolized by a variety of systems. Pseudocholinesterase deficiency can therefore add to unwanted, delayed metabolism of drugs such as procaine.

All these compounds are weak bases and, as such, have two forms, the ionized cation and the un-ionized base. At any one time the relative amount of each will depend on the equilibrium pKa of that particular agent and the pH of the medium it is in:

$$pKa - pH = \log \frac{[\text{cation}]}{[\text{base}]}$$

The significance of this is that it is the cationic, the ionized, form that is the active component in blockade of the sodium channel, while the pharmacologically inactive neutral base is a highly lipid soluble and the form that traverses membranes. As the plasma of tissue pH changes, changes will be seen in the efficacy of the blockade and resulting analgesia. Similarly, by carbonating local anesthetics, inward migration of membrane-permeable CO_2

Table 5–3. Local Anesthetics

Amides	Metabolism site	Anesthesia duration (mins.)	Relative potency	CNS Toxic Dose (mg/kg)
Lidocaine	liver	100	2	6.4
Bupivacaine	liver	175	8	1.6
Prilocaine	liver	100	2	>6
Esters				
Procaine	plasma	50	1	19.2
Tetracaine	plasma	175	8	2.5

Source: Prithvi R.P. *Handbook of Regional Anesthesia.* New York, Churchill Livingstone, 1985.

in preference to impermeable HCO_3 will lower the intercellular pH, increase the proportion of cation, and thereby improve the blockade. The local anesthetics have a range of potencies and durations, and they represent a group of highly studied and characterized drugs which, if well understood by the practitioner and employed with good practical skills, are predictable, efficacious, and safe.

Interestingly, with such potent drugs, allergic reactions are rare and almost entirely confined to the esters. Hence lidocaine and bupivacaine are hardly known to produce such effects.

Topical Method

General anesthesia represents one end of the range of pain control methods. Progressively less invasive methods, including centrally active narcotics and regional analgesia, lead to the other end of the spectrum, where we have methods of pain control that specifically focus on the skin. Since this is the target organ of PWS laser therapy, such specificity of pain control would obviously be ideal.

Cold is one of the oldest agents of analgesia. In Napoleon's retreat from Moscow, Baron Larrey used refrigeration in surgical procedures, and in 1866 an ether spray was used to produce analgesia, superseded by the modern ethyl chloride spray as early as 1890. The mechanism is that of blocking local nerve conduction. Ice bags applied to the skin represent a simple way of producing this effect with a controlled temperature that will not produce skin damage. Histories of cryoglobulinemia or Raynaud's syndrome would be contraindications.

In practice this technique, i.e., application of ice bags, has been found to be very effective in PWS laser therapy. As there seems to be a cumulative effect over time, a 30-minute use prior to the therapy, and then during it, is very helpful. Whereas such an application of cold in normal skin might be associated with vasoconstriction, thereby reducing the target chromophore of the vessels, it seems the ectatic PWS vessels are much less under autonomic control than normal vessels, and hence only minimum effects are seen from this degree of refrigeration.

Topical Local Anesthetics

Although textbooks refer to the ''excellent'' topical properties of certain local anesthetics, these descriptions refer to mucous membrane transport, oral, urethral, and other tissues, but not skin. In fact, the intact skin is normally relatively impermeable to most drugs. Although there has been a long history of attempts to use substances such as DMSO and the electrical augmentation of iontophoresis to improve drug transport through the skin, skin anesthesia by topical application of the local anesthetics has been disappointing up to the last 10 years. Amethocaine, long known to have good absorption characteristics, is currently undergoing a new examination,[8] but its particular toxicity raises problems with its use.

The development of EMLA (eutectic mixture of local anesthetics), a combination of lidocaine and prilocaine, has resulted in a new approach to topical anesthesia. At the time of writing, this product has not been released in the U.S., although it is in widespread use in Europe, particularly for pediatric IV placement, and most of the studies on it are in the European literature.

As EMLA seems to represent a preferred approach to analgesia for PWS laser surgery, current information on it is worth summarizing. Its value, of course, lies in the efficiency of the analgesia it is claimed to produce, and thus the methods by which this is measured are important in evaluating this product or any other technique.

Measuring Analgesia

How good are our analgesia techniques? Because of the individual and subjective nature of pain, measure, and the difficulties with measure, have always loomed large in this field. Clinicians have often relied on ad hoc assessments of analgesia. Yet when there exists a variety of distinct approaches to the alleviation of acute pain, and thereby choice of method arises, it becomes important to have some measure at least of relative efficacy. Attempts to employ ''objective'' parametric measurements, for example, pulse rate, even plasma levels of catecholamines, are not really satisfactory. Other approaches, employing nonparametric measures, have included objective ''behavioral'' scoring and both objective and subjective assessments of pain scoring, often a verbal score, with simple categories of degree of pain.

The most commonly used method is the Visual Analogue Scale (VAS), which, by trial and error, has become standardized to a horizontal 10 cm line with extremes defined as ''No Pain'' and ''Worse Pain Imaginable.'' Effective use of the VAS to produce a reliable, self-reporting measure of pain requires an alert and cooperative patient who is capable of understanding the construct.

The questions that arise when young children are asked to use such self-reporting methods are extensively discussed by Ross and Ross[5] and Lloyd-Thomas.[9] A common approach is to modify the VAS scale either by replacing it entirely with expressive faces or by combining a facial with a purely analogue scale. In addition, it is common practice to supplement whatever self-reporting method is used with parallel objective scoring by the involved clinician and/or a separate observer. Thus in nine trials of the efficacy of EMLA in venipuncture in children,[10–18] only one[11] did not supplement the child's self-scoring with an objective observer's scoring. One study[14] based on 111 children from 1 to 5 years of age did not include self-scoring, but instead used two objective observers. In general, when simple pain scoring methods, typically 4 category verbal scores, were made, they correlated well with VAS scores.

Although day-to-day clinical practice does not call for such assessments on a routine basis, it is important to have good data to support the assessment of new, noninvasive analgesic techniques in children; furthermore, if the practitioner makes sensitive assessment of the child's pain, such an assessment can be assumed to reflect the true pain.

Interestingly, in this same set of studies, the point is made repeatedly that anxiety is a large component of the child's total concept of pain, and that premedication by benzodiazepine, for example, can be an important adjunct to the specific analgesia therapy.

Key clinical features of the pharmacokinetics of this drug are very well summarized in a study by Evers et al.[19] using adult subjects. Analgesia to pin prick was found to depend on both the concentration and duration of application of the cream. While a low concentration, 1.0%, was relatively ineffective, 2.5% and 5% concentrations were associated with excellent analgesia. The 5% concentration has in fact been chosen in the commercially available formulation. Sixty minutes of application under occlusion is required to give a high frequency of painless pin pricks. After removal of the cream the analgesia persists for at least 1 hour; analysis of plasma levels of lidocaine and prilocaine similarly demonstrate that systemic vascular concentrations continue to rise for 2 hours before subsiding.

These parameters have been confirmed by others[20] and have formed the basis for clinical use of the drug for both adults and children. However, variations on these absorption profiles are clearly important and must be considered. With respect to body location, Juhlin et al.[21] demonstrated that when EMLA was applied to the face, absorption, as demonstrated by plasma lidocaine and prilocaine levels, reached over twice the peak level in less than half the time compared with the equivalent uptake from the arm (while still remaining minute fractions of toxic levels). This enhanced absorption through the skin of the face and also the genital area might well be expected, paralleling vascularity.

Similarly, a much more rapid absorption of EMLA through the oral mucous membranes has been established. Holst and Evers[22] showed that only a 5-minute application of 5% EMLA cream to the buccal mucosa produced significant analgesia to pin prick. In addition to location, the condition of the skin must be considered. In the same study cited above, Juhlin et al.[23] examined EMLA on subjects with atopic dermatitis. In this condition, analgesia onset was extremely rapid, 15 minutes, and the therapeutic time window of this analgesia was short, only 15 to 30 minutes. In contrast, in black skin it has been noted[24] that analgesia and presumably absorption are attenuated in comparison to white skin, possibly owing to an increased density in the stratum corneum.

Whereas all the studies noted above relate to adult subjects, it has been common that in the large number of studies in children (10 to 18), a 60-minute application of the cream has been utilized.

Analgesia, of course, is the usual objective of the use of the EMLA cream; but other effects have been noted. The most obvious of these, and noted in almost all the studies, has been a pattern of blanching and then erythema of the skin in some proportion of subjects; this occurs in the area of application of the cream and appears related to the length of time of application. The incidence of this effect varies, probably depending to some extent on the level of precision of reporting protocol. Juhlin[21] initially described the pattern in normal skin as slight blanching in 1 hour, progressing to more pronounced blanching after 2 hours, followed by erythema. By contrast, in atopic skin blanching occurred as rapidly as 1 minute in 40%, was seen in all after 15 minutes, and was succeeded by erythema after 30 to 60 minutes. In the studies in children with 60-minute applications of EMLA, typical incidences were 50% blanching, 5% erythema.[14]

Covino et al.[25] proposed a biphasic response of vasculature to local anesthetics whereby vasoconstriction at low concentrations was followed by vasodilation at higher concentrations; this has been demonstrated by Johns.[26] In all cases these skin changes resolved rapidly with no sequelae and might well be ignored as minor side effects, except that they suggest a much wider spectrum for the mechanisms of action—beyond the direct depolarization of afferent nociceptive fibers—of the local anesthetic ingredients.

Several trials of EMLA have taken place in fields other than acute pain. Ohlsen et al.[27] have shown that EMLA protects the skin from the damaging effects of therapeutic irradiation by inhibiting the normal inflammatory reaction, and they suggest various possibilities for the mechanism: an induced hypovascularity, the known antithrombotic effect of the drugs preventing vascular damage, inhibition of leukocyte mobility, stabilizing effects on the cell membrane, and radical scavenging. Cassuto[28] has shown that EMLA suppresses the eruption of lesions in herpes and postulates inhibition of capillary permeability or interruption of local axonal reflexes involved in the inflammatory response (presumably via substance P).

Pipkorn[29] had previously demonstrated that EMLA cream inhibits the flare but not the wheal response to allergens, including histamine, and also concluded that a distinct role of the local anesthetics is to block the axonal reflex that is at least partially responsible for this flare effect.

It has also been noted that pruritis, a phenomenon thought to utilize the same nerve fiber pathways as acute pain, but distinct in its mechanisms, is also suppressed by EMLA.[30]

Thus, there is a great deal of experimental evidence that the actions of the local anesthetics in EMLA probably involve various mechanisms that together suppress the several distinct and unpleasant components associated with laser-induced trauma, i.e., mechanical shock, fast pin-prick pain, second burning pain, wheal and flare inflammation, and itching.

Depth of Penetration of EMLA

The time-dependent characteristics first of the onset, and then of the increasing completeness of analgesia to skin trauma, suggest a progressive penetration from the surface through layers of the skin, although this simplistic model is probably complicated by distinct rates of onset of nerve blockade of different nociceptor fiber types (unmyelinated before myelinated) at the same level.

In some of the clinical application studies involving split-skin harvesting[31–33] and radial artery cannulation[34] as well as the most common application, venipuncture, there have been attempts to correlate different modalities of sensation with depth of penetration of the EMLA cream. Unfortunately, there is insufficient information about the density and distribution of distinct nociceptor and other nerve types in the different layers of the skin to support such correlations; in general, only one study[35] has specifically attempted to establish the characteristics of EMLA's depth penetration by using a measured trauma. Based on pin-prick trauma the investigators describe a linear time/depth of penetration characteristic: 3 mm analgesia depth at 60 minutes extending to 5 mm at 120 minutes.

Although this is useful, pin-prick pain is not necessarily the same as laser surgery pain. The pulsed dye laser treatment of PWS induces a trauma of a distinct type with a penetration depth down to fat. Two published studies[36,37] show that EMLA is efficacious to dermatologic lasers in adults; our own work[38] demonstrates that in children this cream also works and is a rational part of the approach to PWS therapy in children.

EMLA Side Effects: Methemoglobinemia

The skin blanching and erythema associated with the application of EMLA for extended periods, while occurring in some patients, is self-limiting and appears to be a minor side effect. The systemic uptake of the local anesthetics from normal skin application is insignificant, with resulting plasma levels being a minute fraction of those toxic levels correlated with cardiac or cerebral effects. Prilocaine, however, has been known for many years to associate with methemoglobinemia. Jakobson et al.[39] describe a case history of a 12-week-old baby who, after an excessively long application of EMLA (5 hours), developed hypoxia secondary to methemoglobinemia; the condition was reversed by intravenous methylene blue. Any methemoglobin formed in everyday life is normally reduced to hemoglobin by the enzyme NADH-methemoglobin reductase. Neonates are deficient in this enzyme by about 50%, and develop adult levels only over the first 3 months of life.[40] Occasionally more serious congenital deficiencies occur, and certain drugs, notably trimethoprim-sulfamethoxazole, can contribute to reduced enzyme activity and methemoglobinemia. Methemoglobin levels can peak up to 24 hours after application[41]; so, although such levels in studied groups of children[40,41] are low, it is important to take an accurate history and use EMLA within safe guidelines. Engberg et al.[40] define safe guidelines as 3 months or older, no medication with a known inducing agent, and less than 2 grams of cream on an area of less than 16 cm^2, with a maximum application time of 4 hours.

Summary

The approach to the handling of pain in dermatologic laser surgery, as in any surgery, is a question for the individual clinician. Some may choose general anesthesia for its obvious specific advantages and thereby accept its attendant costs and complications. Others may choose minimally invasive techniques; but even in this latter circumstance, the unusual and unexpected can always occur. Hence it is prudent to know in great detail the pharmacology of any drug administered, even drugs as ''safe'' as the local anesthetics, and also to have the equipment, skills, and procedures to deal with any emergency.

In one clinic where we have worked, while we have been equipped and prepared to offer the full variety of techniques, we found local digital nerve blocks indicated in only a handful of cases. For the rest of the first 10,000-plus treatments, we have found both adequate and appropriate the use of topical methods of analgesia (cold and local anesthetic) supplemented by light awake sedation in a selected number of children. No cases of nausea and vomiting, prolonged recovery, or other complications occurred. Two cases of seizures in known epileptics, easily treated, underlined the need to be responsive to any emergency. Of course, this approach does demand the ability of the clinician to handle fears, anxieties, and occasional discomfort.

References

1. Campbell JN, et al. Peripheral neural mechanisms of nociception. *In* Textbook of Pain. 2nd Ed. Edited by Wall P, Melzack R. New York, Churchill Livingston, 1989.
2. Talman B, et al. Location of portwine stains and the likelihood of ophthalmic and/or central nervous system complications. Pediatrics 87:3, 1991.
3. Strempel H. Circadian cycles of epicritic and propathic pain threshold. J Inter-disciplinary Cycle Res 8:276, 1977.
4. Wolff BB. Behavioral measurement of human pain. *In* The Psychology of Pain. Edited by Strenbach R. New York. Raven Press, 1978, pp 129.
5. Ross DM, Ross SA. Childhood Pain: Current Issues, Research, and Management. Chicago. Donnelley & Sons, 1988.
6. Mittwoch T, et al. The influence of warning signal timing and cognitive preparation on the aversiveness of electric shock. Pain 42:373, 1990.
7. Prithvi RP. Handbook of Regional Anesthesia. New York, Churchill Livingstone, 1988.
8. Coley S. Anesthesia of the skin (editorial). Br J Anaesth 62:4, 1989.
9. Lloyd-Thomas AR. Pain management in pediatric patients. Br J Anaesth 64:85, 1990.
10. Maunuksela EL, Korpela R. Double-blind evaluation of a lignocaine-prilocaine cream (EMLA) in children. Br J Anaesth 58:1242, 1986.
11. Hallen B, Olsson GL, Uppfeldt A. Pain-free venipuncture. Anaesthesia 39:969, 1984.
12. Manner T, et al. Reduction of pain at venous cannulation in children with a eutectic mixture of lidocaine and prilocaine (EMLA cream): comparison with placebo cream and no local premedication. Acta Anaesthesiol Scand 31:735, 1987.
13. Soliman IR, et al. Comparison of the analgesic effects of EMLA (eutectic mixture of local anesthetics) to intradermal lidocaine infiltration prior to venous cannulation in unpremedicated children. Anesthesiology 68:804, 1988.
14. Hopkins CS, et al. Pain-free injection in infants. Anaesthesia 43:198, 1988.
15. Cooper CM, et al. EMLA cream reduces the pain of venipuncture in children. Eur J Anaesth 4:441, 1987.
16. Hallen B, et al. Does lidocaine-prilocaine cream permit painfree insertion of IV catheters in children? Anesthesiology 57:340, 1982.
17. Clarke S, Radford M. Topical anaesthesia for venipuncture. J Br Paed Assoc 61:1132, 1986.
18. Wahlstedt C, et al. Lignocaine-prilocaine cream reduces venipuncture pain. Lancet 11:106, 1984.
19. Evers H, Von Dardel O, Juhlin L, Ohlsen L, Vinnars E. Dermal effects of compositions based on the eutectic mixture of lignocaine and prilocaine. Br J Anaesth 57:997, 1985.
20. Maddi R, Concepcion M, Horrow JC, et al. Evaluation of a new cutaneous topical anesthesia preparation. Regional Anesthesia 15:109, 1990.
21. Juhlin L, Hagglund G, Evers H. Absorption of lidocaine and prilocaine after application of a eutectic mixture of local anesthetics (EMLA) on normal and diseased skin. Acta Derm Venereol 69:18, 1989.
22. Holst A, Evers H. Experimental studies of new topical anaesthetics on the oral mucosa. Swed Dent J 9:185, 1985.
23. Juhlin L, Rollman O. Vascular effects of a local anesthetic in atopic dermatitis. Acta Derm Venereol 64:439, 1984.
24. Hymes JA, Spraker MK. Racial differences in the effectiveness of a topically applied mixture of local anesthetics. Regional Anaesthesia 11:11, 1986.
25. Covino B, Vasallo H. Local Anesthetics: Mechanism of Action and Clinical Use. New York, Grune & Stratton, 1976.
26. Johns RA, et al. Lidocaine constricts or dilates rat arteroids in a dose dependent manner. Anesthesiology 61:4, 1984.
27. Ohlsen L, Evers H, Segerstrom K, et al. Local anaesthetics modifying the dermal response of irradiation: an experimental study. Acta Oncol 26:467–475, 1987.
28. Cassuto J. Topical local anaesthetics and herpes simplex. Lancet 1:100, 1989.
29. Pipkorn U, Andersson M. Topical dermal anaesthesia inhibits the flare but not the wheal response to allergen and histamine in the skin-prick test. Clin Allergy 17:307, 1987.
30. Shuttleworth D, Hill S, Marks R, Connelly DM. Relief of experimentally induced pruritus with a novel eutectic mixture of local anaesthetic agents. Br J Dermatol 119:535, 1988.

31. Ohlsen L, Englesson S, Evers H. An anaesthetic lidocaine/prilocaine cream (EMLA) for epicutaneous application tested for cutting split skin grafts. Scand J Plast Reconstr Surg. 19:201–209, 1985. *And* Scand J Plast Surg 41:533, 1988.
32. Strombeck JO, Uggla M, Lillieborg S. Percutaneous anaesthesia with a lidocaine-prilocaine cream (EMLA) for cutting split-skin grafts. Eur J Plast Surg 11:49, 1988.
33. Goodacre TEE, Sanders R, Watts DA, Stoker M. Split skin grafting using topical local anaesthesia (EMLA): a comparison with infiltrated anaesthesia. Br J Plast Surg 41:533, 1988.
34. Russell GN, Desmond MJ, Fox MA. Local anesthesia for radial artery cannulation: a comparison of a lidocaine-prilocaine emulsion and lidocaine infiltration. J Cardiothorac Anesth 2:309, 1988.
35. Bjerring P, Arendt-Nielsen L. Depth and duration of skin analgesia to needle insertion after epicutaneous EMLA cream application. (In press)
36. Arendt-Nielsen L, Bjerring P. Laser-induced pain for evaluation of local analgesia: a comparison of topical application (EMLA) and local injection (lidocaine). Anesth Analg 67:115, 1988.
37. Lanigan SW, Cotterhill JA. Use of a lidocaine-prilocaine cream as an analgesic in dye laser treatment of port-wine stains. Lasers Med Sci 2:72, 1987.
38. Tan OT, Stafford TJ. EMLA for laser treatment of portwine stains in children. Lasers Surg Med (In press.) 1992.
39. Jakobson B, Nilsson A. Methemoglobinemia associated with a prilocaine-lidocaine cream and trimethoprim-sulphamethoxazole. A case report. Acta Anaesthesiol Scand 29:453, 1985.
40. Engberg G, Danielson K, Henneberg S, Nilsson A. Plasma concentrations of prilocaine and lidocaine and methaemoglobin formation in infants after epicutaneous application of a 5% lidocaine-prilocaine cream (EMLA). Acta Anaesthesiol Scand 31:624, 1987.
41. Frayling IM, et al. Methaemoglobinaemia in children treated with prilocaine lidocaine cream. Br J Med 301:153, 1990.

Chapter 6   Pulsed Dye Laser Treatment of Adult Port-Wine Stains

Oon Tian Tan

Adults with port-wine stain (PWS) present to the clinician for laser treatment with untreated lesions, having had test sites performed, or with entire lesions treated using other modalities. Treatment modalities used to remove PWS birthmarks include:

- X-ray irradiation
- Tattooing
- Surgery and skin graft
- Cryosurgery
- Electrocautery
- Dermabrasion
- Other laser treatments,
     e.g., argon, CO_2, Nd:YAG

Whereas the pediatric population generally present for laser treatment with a relatively uniform type of birthmark (pale pink, macular), adult patients with port-wine stains have distinct patterns at presentation. Adults not only have had their PWS for a longer time, but in some instances many have already had their birthmarks treated by other modalities such as those listed above. (See Fig. 6–1.)

The consequences of having a PWS for decades rather than months or even a few years are often evident in the adult patients. In general, the affected lesions have enlarged from the initial, infantile presentation in parallel with the normal process of growth, so that an adult lesion has a larger surface area. Other processes also take place. The sequelae of maturation of a previously untreated PWS include progressive darkening of the birthmark, hypertrophy of the affected site, and in some cases development of nodules within the PWS (Figs. 6–2, 6–3). The latter often bleed when traumatized, requiring surgery to stop the bleeding.

Clinical symptoms of "compression" of adjacent dermal structures—such as peripheral nerves, particularly in confined compartments, i.e., limbs, hands, fingers—through progressive ectasia of the abnormal PWS blood vessels can also be problematic (see Chapter 14).

In cases when the PWS has previously been treated, the results of the various treatment modalities are often evident. Such results include the

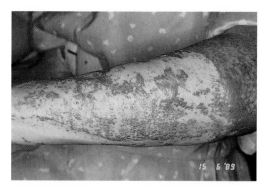

A

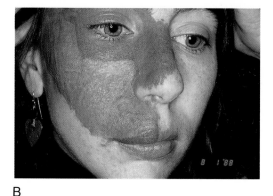

B

Fig. 6–1. *A.* Postsurgically excised and grafted port-wine stain on the left arm. Note that the PWS vessels have regrown through the grafted skin. *B.* Postargon laser treated PWS on the right side of the face. Note that the periorbital and nasal PWS skin were not treated using this laser for fear of inducing scarring.

presence of both atrophic and hypertrophic scar formation, abnormal pigmentation (hypo- and/or hyperpigmentation), and incomplete clearance of the birthmark itself (see Fig. 6–4).

Reasons Why Adults With PWS Seek Treatment

It is generally assumed of individuals who have reached adulthood with birth defects that "they have learned to live with their abnormality." Such a presumption is often incorrect. In many individuals, the wish to have the lesion removed has increased rather than diminished over time. Rather, these people have had to live with their defects because their own highly motivated and extensive investigations often have revealed to them that no effective treatments with minimal adverse effects were available, or that the current treatment modalities appeared "experimental" (techniques and hardware appeared incompletely developed) and without long-term followup. Because of all this, the results were regarded as unpredictable and, in many instances, the adverse effects resulting from these treatments were deemed to exceed the benefits; or, alternatively, in those instances in which test sites were performed on the PWS using other modalities, results were actually seen to be ineffective or less than satisfactory (Fig. 6–4A,B).

Because the claimed and promised results from the various treatment modalities have, until recently, been disappointing, such experiences have

Fig. 6–2. Mature PWS which has produced hypertrophy of the affected side. Note that nodules have started to develop in the maturing PWS.

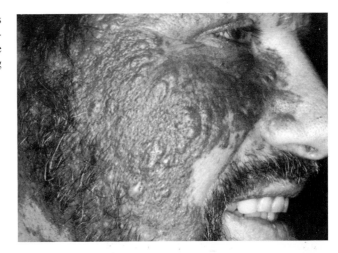

Fig. 6–3. Change in PWS color and morphology in the same individual from infancy to young adulthood. *A.* At infancy. *B.* At 4 years. *C.* At 10 years. *D.* At 15 years.

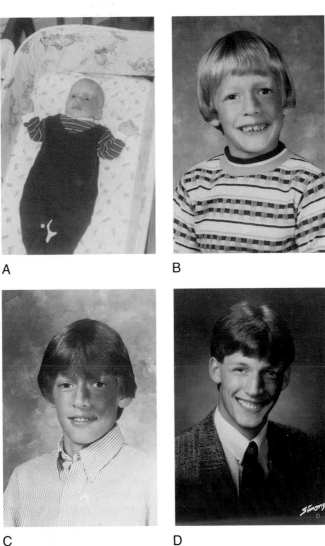

A

B

C

D

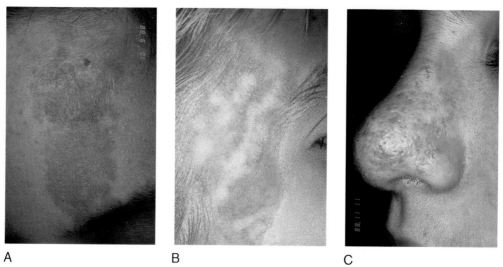

A   B   C

Fig. 6–4. *A.* Hypertrophic scar which developed after exposure to the argon laser. *B.* Atrophic scar following argon laser treatment. Note the hypopigmentation which also resulted from this treatment. *C.* Less severe scar resulting from argon laser treatments. Note that residual PWS vessels are still present in the laser-exposed site.

tended to make PWS subjects skeptical, apprehensive, and confused. It is therefore not surprising that these have been the reactions when a new treatment is introduced into the therapeutic arena. Many are afraid to be optimistic and, in general, have found it difficult to evaluate objectively the effectiveness of new treatment modalities. The patient's apprehension, when accompanied by the overenthusiastic recommendations of some investigators, leads to a compounded confusion. Despite all this, PWS subjects still continue to seek and explore new treatments, always hoping that a treatment will eventually be developed that will erase their birthmarks without producing too many side effects.

The most common reasons why adults with PWS seek treatment for their birthmark include a change in the lesion itself and a change in life style.

Change In The Lesion Itself. As individuals mature, PWS tends to darken, increase in bulkiness (hypertrophy), and, in some, develop nodules within the birthmark (Fig. 6–2). Such changes, occurring gradually over time, make the birthmark more conspicuous and less easy to camouflage with makeup; when hypertrophy occurs, underlying structures such as nerves can become compressed, producing pain and other symptoms. Typically, this is seen in an arm and/or hand, where hypertrophy of the affected area may not only produce pain but also restrict hand movement owing to enlargement of the fingers. Similarly, architectural effects involving the nose and periorbital areas are seen in compression of the lacrimal duct by the PWS, producing blockage of the ducts and constant lacrimation.

Change In Life Style. Individuals often seek treatment when significant life events loom, for example, a wedding or a career change. Some, particularly those greater than 40 years old, seek treatment because they find the elaborately camouflaging of their birthmark with makeup has become time consuming and tedious. Others, through failing sight, find it progressively more difficult to apply their makeup on their birthmarks. There are also those who are dissatisfied with results from previous treatment modalities and want their lesion "lightened" or improved.

Psychologic Impact of the Birthmark

Although there is controversy within the medical profession regarding the degree of psychologic impact that PWS birthmarks have on individuals, our own experience has been that the lesion almost invariably involves a large psychologic challenge in affected individuals. At the same time, we have been impressed by the different ways individuals (adults and families) have emotionally handled this defect.

Superficially, individuals with PWS have tended to fall into two categories: those who appear "unaffected" by the birthmark, and those whose lives have been obviously altered and constrained. However, despite this polar presentation of psychologic accommodation, a much wider spectrum of common themes of experience is revealed as these patients are given the opportunity to discuss their feelings and reactions when presenting for laser treatments, especially as the birthmark becomes progressively lighter with successive pulsed dye laser treatments.

Many recall their feeling of *isolation,* most vivid in childhood and still persisting into adulthood. They describe being isolated from their friends because of their appearance, and in some instances experiencing even frank revulsion from their peers. In addition, the constant stare and questions from strangers have been stressful. With children, remarks made are often accusatory and directed at the parents. Children are often questioned, "What happened to your face?" People refer to "the burn on your face," or "the grape juice," and in some instances parents have even been accused of child abuse. The public, in general, appears to be intolerant of physical differences and anomalies, and even the presumably "harmless" inquisitiveness of the individuals can be hurtful. Remarks made are often thoughtless and hurtful. Few realize what long-term effects their remarks have had upon the individuals with PWS and their families (see Chapter 14).

Some parents feel responsible and are guilt-ridden for their child's birth defect. Many question whether events occurring during their pregnancy (such as trauma) or ingestion of certain foods (like red wine) could have produced the birthmark.

Blame, the stigma of being different, isolation, frustration, anger, and the feeling of being "emotionally trapped" have been some of the feelings described by these patients. Interestingly, individuals have dealt with these feelings in different ways. Some have used them as a challenge to excel in their adult and professional lives. Others, burdened by the birthmark, have in their feeling of isolation become introverted. Whichever group the patient falls into, most have undergone significant change during the treatment course. It has been fascinating to watch the personality changes that have accompanied the gradual lightening and disappearance of the PWS with successive pulsed dye laser treatments.

Psychologic Effect of Pulsed Dye Laser Treatment

The change in personality of individual PWS subjects as the birthmark progressively lightens and eventually disappears has been remarkable. Sad, introverted, self-conscious individuals lose their frown, becoming happier and more outgoing. Smiles replace grimaces. Upright, confident postures replace downcast, stooped statures. Improved self-image and confidence have manifested in several of these individuals. Several, especially young adults, have dieted and lost weight as the birthmarks have cleared. The dramatic changes in body and self-image have, in some cases, also been accompanied by significant changes in these individuals' lives, including an upward movement in their career goals.

Children previously "protected" by their parents, always conscious of being different, have had to learn and understand that these differences no longer exist once their birthmark clears; they have had to learn to live and be like their siblings and peers, no longer having the excuse to retreat and hide behind their PWS. Can this change be problematic? Only those children who have made this transition and experienced the impact of this change can address the issue. Nor is this situation confined to the affected child. Commonly, the entire family, parents and siblings, consciously or not, have structured themselves to the PWS individual and have had to reaccommodate their family relationships.

Although happiness and improved self-image dominate towards the end of the pulsed dye laser treatment program, despondency and doubt can dominate in the middle of the program. It may be particularly difficult during this stage when progress is slow, improvement is progressively less dramatic, and treatment visits seem endless. It is tempting at such times for patients to become despondent and either stop treatment or seek treatment elsewhere. Physicians may feel pressured by these reactions and decisions, often responding by modifying the laser treatment program. Hastening the treatment program by increasing either the number of return visits or the laser fluence can be harmful. It is critical that patients be given a perspective of what progress has occurred in the birthmark, what further improvements can be expected, and how the treatment program will proceed.

Assessment and Treatment Plan

As has been discussed, adults with PWS presenting for treatment differ from their pediatric counterparts in several ways. Many adults present having had their birthmark treated by other modalities. Therefore, a careful history of previous treatments is important. The details of previous treatments will not only influence the laser parameters to be used in the dye laser treatment protocol, but also should alert the physician to be watchful for potential problems, e.g., malignancy in x-irradiated skin and/or underlying structures.[1]

Previously Untreated Port-wine Stains

Adults with PWS presenting for pulsed dye laser treatment often present with birthmarks of different colors (dark red to purple) and of various sizes. They can range in size from a few square centimeters to lesions involving an entire half of a face, a limb, or even the whole body. Not only are these lesions darker than those presenting in childhood (Figs. 6–2, 6–3), but they are often raised and have nodules developing within them, the latter bleeding when traumatized. Because of these differences, the laser parameters needed for treating these dark, thickened, elevated PWS lesions in adults will differ from those used for children (see Chapter 7).

Previously Treated PWS

Previous treatment modalities can involve any one of those listed at the start of this chapter. In general, each of these treatment modalities will have altered or damaged structures in both the epidermis and the dermis. The degree of injury potentially induced in the PWS will depend upon the modality used and the expertise of the therapist. Previously treated PWS range from those that have been scarred and have an architecture grossly altered by the treatments (Fig. 6–4A,B) to others that are apparently less affected (Fig. 6–4C).

It is particularly important for the physician to spend time discussing in great detail what the outcome of the pulsed dye laser treatment on the PWS will be, as well as the patient's expectations of the therapy. Many patients—through enthusiastic recommendations of physicians, health care professionals, and other patients who are familiar and experienced with the new laser technique—often come with unrealistically high expectations of a ''cure'' for their birthmark. In many instances the patient believes that the laser will not only remove the birthmark but also replace the areas of scarring and abnormal pigmentation with normal-appearing skin pigment and complete removal of the birthmark itself. Unless a realistic prognosis and description of what the patient can expect after the pulsed dye laser treatment are carefully and clearly outlined and discussed, the patients are likely to be disappointed, frustrated, and angry.

It is important at the initial visit to inform the patient of two points. First, any hypopigmentation which has resulted from previous treatments will be revealed when the underlying port-wine vessels making the birthmark red are destroyed by the pulsed dye laser (Fig. 6–5). Second, the hyperpigmentation

Fig. 6–5. *A*. Pre pulsed dye laser treated but post argon laser induced hyper- and hypopigmentation in the laser-exposed PWS. ***B*.** Hypopigmentation in argon laser treated PWS is unmasked following pulsed dye laser treatment of the birthmark.

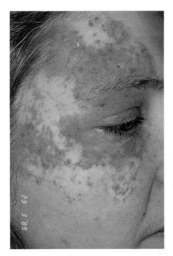
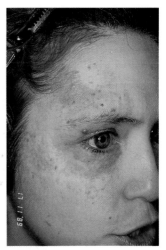

A   B

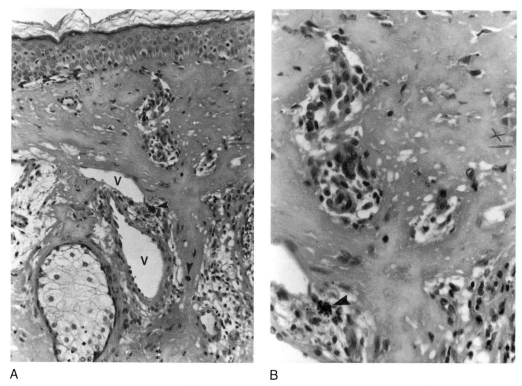

A   B

Fig. 6–6. *A.* Light microscopy of PWS skin showing the presence of intact vessels (V) lying beyond the papillary dermis. *B.* Melanophages (arrow heads) in the dermis following exposure of the area to the argon laser.

inherent in many previously treated sites will also remain and be unaffected by the pulsed dye laser. This will occur when the hyperpigmentation is due to melanophages trapped in the dermis, and not the hemosiderin that was previously postulated (Fig. 6–6) in these situations.

Laser Parameters for Previously Treated PWS

Pulsed dye laser parameters needed to treat the birthmark will depend upon the severity and extent of damage induced by the previous treatment modality used in the PWS. In cases where scarring is clearly evident, higher fluences than those used to treat untreated PWS will be required to reach the abnormal PWS vessels lying beyond the zone of the scar tissue. The increase in fluence should compensate for the change in optical properties of the dermis and allow the laser beam to penetrate through the scar tissue to reach the abnormal PWS vessels beyond.

Not only should the treatment fluence be increased (usually by 0.5 to 1.0 J/cm^2) but the patient also should be warned that progress will be slow and the treatment program itself will be prolonged.

Tattooed PWS

PWS previously tattooed with skin-colored pigment in attempts to camouflage the redness of the birthmark will also affect the fluence needed to lighten the birthmark. The problems encountered with treatment of these birthmarks will include:

1. The need for a higher fluence (between 0.5 and 1.0 J/cm^2) to effectively lighten the birthmark.
2. The formation of vesicles and, in some instances, even small blisters within hours to days of laser treatment. The working assumption here is that the tattoo pigment lying near the dermal-epidermal junction (DEJ), and thus anatomically more superficially than the PWS vessels, will competitively absorb the laser energy.
3. Percutaneous elimination of the tattoo pigment during the healing period of the laser-treated PWS. Areas where this has occurred have, in some cases, become impetiginized, requiring systemic antibiotic treatment.
4. Accentuation of the pigmentary and textural changes following lightening of the PWS (Fig. 6–7).
5. Inability to completely erase the PWS (Fig. 6–7B).

Knowing that some, if not all, of these events could occur, it is important that these issues be discussed with the patient prior to commencement of

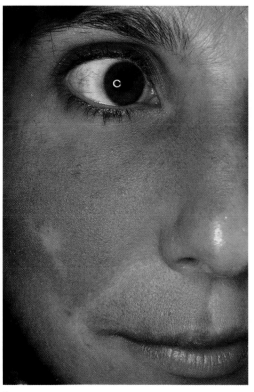

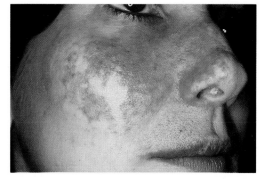

B

Fig. 6–7. *A.* PWS on the lip that was previously treated by tattooing pigment into the area to camouflage the abnormal blood vessels. Note the textural change in the skin following the tattooing. *B.* Incomplete clearance of the tattooed PWS even after multiple pulsed dye laser exposures. Note that the tattooed skin has a different texture and the area still has a significant amount of pigment in the skin.

A

treatment. By doing this, the patients are prepared for the outcome, and expectations become more realistic.

Electrocautery and Cryosurgically Treated PWS

The most striking change in a port-wine stain treated with either electrocautery or cryosurgery has been the textural change of the treated site (Fig. 6–8).

The rationale for using these modalities in the past for "erasing" PWS was to physically destroy the superficial PWS blood vessels. Unfortunately, because it was impossible to control the extent of damage induced by either treatment modality, this resulted in nonspecific injury of the treated site. The adverse effects induced in many cases were greater than the therapeutic benefits achieved. Again, because of the extent of injury induced by these treatment modalities, changes in the skin texture accompanied by loss of epidermal pigment will be amplified when the underlying PWS blood vessels are destroyed by the pulsed dye laser. All of these changes will be accentuated when the PWS is lightened by the pulsed dye laser.

Argon Laser Treated PWS

There has been controversy regarding the effect of the argon laser on PWS. The controversy has centered around the extent of thermal injury induced by the argon laser and how this injury heals.

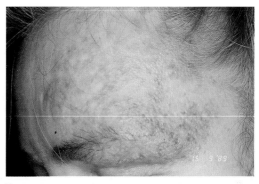

B

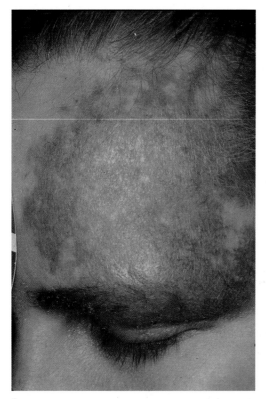

A

Fig. 6–8. *A*. PWS following multiple electrocautery treatments over many years. Within the PWS are many areas of marked textural and color change. ***B*.** Post electrocautery treated PWS that was subsequently treated using the pulsed dye laser. Note that although a large proportion of the PWS has cleared following dye laser treatments, there are many areas which are still present. Note that the scarring, textural and color changes induced by electrocautery are unmasked.

The argon laser has been effective for lightening and/or clearing "mature" PWS (Chap. 4). Carruth, van Gemert, and Shakespeare discuss the indications and contraindications for the argon laser in Chapter 4. They claim that it has been difficult to compare response of PWS to argon laser treatment because of the lack of objective assessment in the various studies published.

In spite of these difficulties, it is now generally accepted by most that the argon laser does indeed induce nonspecific thermal injury in skin, the extent being dependent upon the expertise of the therapist.[2] Because of this, the injury induced can vary from minimal loss of skin markings to hypertrophic/atrophic scar formation (Fig. 6–4).

A study was recently performed by Alster et al.[3] using histology, optical profilometry, and clinical assessment to: (a) examine differences in argon- and nonargon-treated PWS skin using these three parameters; and (b) establish how the argon-treated PWS was affected by subsequent treatment using the pulsed dye laser. This study demonstrated two main findings. First, the argon laser destroyed only the abnormal PWS vessels in the superficial papillary dermis, leaving the ectatic PWS vessels completely intact in the mid and reticular dermis. Second, the skin markings were indeed altered by argon laser exposure, loss of skin markings being clearly evident in argon-irradiated PWS skin as shown in Figure 6–4. These clinical and histologic findings were substantiated by profilometric measurements, showing clear differences between argon laser irradiated and normal skin. Also demonstrated in the study of Alster et al. was the change in the clinical, histologic, and profilometric measurements of argon laser irradiated PWS skin following multiple pulsed dye laser exposures (Figs. 6–4, 6–6, 6–9, 6–10).

In summary, this study not only demonstrated that it was possible to destroy the ectatic PWS vessels lying beyond the argon-altered dermis, but also found that the scar tissue induced by the argon laser, in some cases, was then affected by subsequent pulsed dye laser exposure of these sites. In spite of these "improvements," it must be remembered that neither the loss of epidermal pigment nor the presence of hyperpigmentation can be altered by the pulsed dye laser.

Fig. 6–9. Mould and profilometry of argon laser treated skin. Note that the tracing of the profile measured across this area is "flatter" than that shown in Figure 6–11.

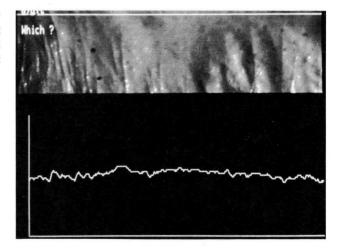

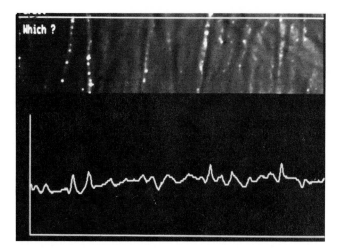

Fig. 6–10. Post dye laser treated PWS profilometry. Note that the skin texture more closely approximates that of normal skin.

Treatment Progress

Immediately After Treatment

Patients should be warned that there will be a blue-gray discoloration of the skin immediately following laser irradiation, darkening to being almost black over the next 24 hours. This discoloration will last for between 10 to 14 days, after which time the treated areas will appear red. Subsequently, fading or lightening of the PWS should be evident over the next 2 to 4 weeks.

Post-treatment Hyperpigmentation

Certain parts of the body appear to be more susceptible to developing hyperpigmentation than others. These include the "fleshy" parts of the cheeks, infraorbital parts of the face, distal parts of the upper limbs, and the whole of both lower limbs.

Darkly pigmented individuals (skin Types IV and V—see Table 3–3), including those who are tanned, are also more likely to develop hyperpigmentation of the laser-treated sites.

In almost all of these instances, the hyperpigmentation should fade and the skin color should return to normal over the next 8 to 12 weeks.

Hyperpigmentation observed at the followup clinic should prompt the clinician either to reduce the laser fluence and/or request that the individual be protected from the sun with the use of PABA-free sunscreens SPF #15 and upwards. In general, it is recommended that *all* patients enrolled for laser treatment use sunscreens throughout the year, both winter and summer.

Post-treatment Hypopigmentation

Hypopigmentation of pulsed dye laser irradiated sites can occur in those with darkly pigmented (both ethnic and sun induced) skin as well as those with very fair Type I skin.

Hypopigmentation, in the presence of normal skin texture and in the absence of scar formation, is often temporary. The hypopigmented areas should, in general, tan normally once the area is re-exposed to the sun when treatment is completed. If, however, hypopigmentation is accompanied by changes in skin texture and/or other signs of scar formation, this loss of pigment is more likely to be permanent. Such damage is often the result of widespread nonspecific damage of pigmented as well as nonpigmented epidermal and dermal cells.

Number of Laser Treatments

The number of treatments required to clear the PWS will depend on the following factors:

- Location of the PWS
- Maturation of the PWS: color, thickness, and degree of hypertrophy of the lesion
- Age of the patient
- Prior treatment of the PWS, e.g., laser, electrocautery

Location of the PWS. A port-wine stain located in certain parts of the body requires more treatments than a PWS in others. Those areas requiring more laser treatments include the cheek (particularly the medial half), sides of the nose, upper lip, chin, forearms and hands, buttocks, and lower limbs.

By contrast, the forehead, temples, lateral half of the face, periorbital areas, ear lobes, neck, shoulders, and chest respond with fewer treatments using the pulsed dye laser. Because these areas usually clear fastest, patients and physicians become frustrated when other areas, especially those noted above, fail to clear at the same rate. The tendency when this occurs is to "turn up the fluence." This can often lead to loss of pigment and scar formation, especially when unnecessarily high fluences (greater than 8 J/cm^2 in previously untreated lesions) are used.

Therefore, when treating a large PWS involving different parts of the body, it must be remembered that the rate of response to the pulsed dye laser will vary according to the anatomic site-to-site variation.

Clinical assessment, experience, and skill in manipulating the appropriate fluences to clear these lesions are required at this stage.

Maturation of the PWS. PWSs as they mature can and often will change in color, from pale pink in infancy to dark purple in adulthood (Fig. 6–3). In addition, they can also change by becoming bulky and elevated (Fig. 6–2). It is likely that all these changes, including hypertrophy of the affected side, are the result of the progressive ectasia of the PWS blood vessels. All these changes make the mature PWS more difficult and more challenging to treat.

The dark, hypertrophied, elevated PWS will require not only significantly more laser treatments to eradicate the lesion, but also more skill on the part of the laser therapist in manipulating the laser fluence to effectively destroy the deep dermal ectatic PWS blood vessels.

Age of the Patient. The ability to selectively destroy the ectatic PWS blood vessels without injuring healthy adjacent structures such as dermal collagen has provided, in contrast to previous recommendations derived from experience with the argon laser,[4,5] a means for treating PWS in the very young.[6,7] In fact, unlike with the argon laser, age is now no longer a reason for withholding laser treatment from children; instead, there are very good reasons why children should commence treatment as soon as possible (see Chapter 7).

It is hoped that early treatment of their PWS will enable those born with these devastating birthmarks to live normal lives instead of having to bear the stigma and burden of these lesions all their lives.

Of course, the fact that pulsed dye laser treatment is currently being advocated particularly for children does not preclude adults from being treated. Adult PWS will respond as well to this treatment modality, provided that the pulsed dye laser beam can reach the vessels to destroy them.[8-10] Again, because the vessels are larger, and the involved area is larger and hypertrophied, more laser treatments are required to lighten and/or clear these lesions.

Prior Treatment of the PWS. See Chapter 3.

Port-Wine Stain Responses to the Pulsed Dye Laser

The pulsed dye laser (577 to 585 nm) has been used to successfully clear PWS in adults as well as in children.[6-10] Good results have been achieved in adults despite criticisms that injury induced by the pulsed dye laser was ''too vascular-specific to destroy the mature, purple, hypertrophic PWS's'' (Fig. 6–11). The most significant differences between pulsed dye laser treatment of children and that of adults have been that: (a) more treatments are required in adults; (b) the range of treatment fluences used for adults is often greater (between 6.25 and 8.00 J/cm^2) than that used for children (between 6.00 and 7.00 J/cm^2); (c) a wider range of fluences needs to be used on different parts of the PWS in adults; and (d) treatment programs for adults tend to be more protracted. Of course, these generalizations are based upon the fact that the color is deeper and the size of the lesion itself as well as the vessels within it are significantly larger than in children.[11]

Of interest is the fact that the hypertrophy apparent in the birthmark disappears as the PWS lightens with successive treatment, becoming normal

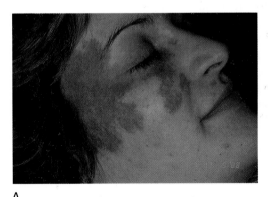
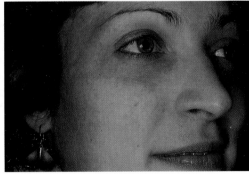

A   B

Fig. 6–11. *A.* Mature PWS on the right side of the face, before pulsed dye laser treatment. *B.* After pulsed dye laser treatment; note the laser-treated skin is indistinguishable in color from normal adjacent skin.

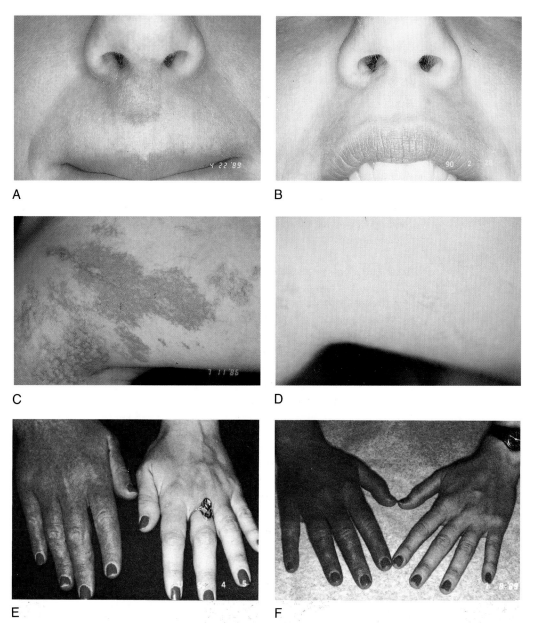

Fig. 6–12. *A.* Pre dye laser treatment of a PWS on the frenulum. *B.* Post dye laser treatment. *C.* Pre dye laser treatment of PWS partly on the thigh, extending onto the leg. *D.* Post dye laser treatment. *E.* Pre dye laser treatment of PWS involving the hand and fingers. *F.* Post dye laser treatment. Note the reduction color of the PWS as well as the size of the fingers, particularly around the knuckles, following multiple pulsed dye laser treatments. Also note that the treated skin texture approximates that of normal skin.

in color and texture as well as returning to its normal anatomic contour at the end of treatment (Fig. 6–11).

The pulsed dye laser has also been successful in treating PWS at sites which were previously contraindicated for treatment by the argon and CO_2 lasers because of the risk of scarring or poor response (Fig. 6–12). Such sites include the upper lip, around the nares, and limbs.

Despite good results with minimal adverse effects associated with the use of the pulsed dye laser for the treatment of PWS in adults, this laser is not the "cure all" for all vascular birthmarks. There are lesions in which the vessels are so large and so deep that few treatment modalities will be effective for altering the birthmark.

Port-Wine Stain and Its Relationship to Other Cutaneous Lesions

Certain observations have been made during the course of PWS treatment using the pulsed dye laser regarding the distribution and behavior of other cutaneous lesions such as acne vulgaris and chickenpox. Although anecdotal, these observations are interesting and worth a note because they could give clues to the pathogenesis of these skin conditions.

Acne and Port-Wine Stains. It has been observed in a few teenage patients with facial PWS and acne that the acne lesions are present on all parts of the face except in the area of the PWS (Fig. 6–13). As the PWS lesions have cleared with successive pulsed dye laser treatments, however, the acne lesions have appeared in those areas previously occupied by the birthmark.

Port-Wine and Chickenpox Lesions. Many parents whose children with PWS have developed varicella have reported the absence or sparsity of chickenpox lesions within the untreated or partially treated birthmark. It has also been reported that chickenpox lesions have appeared, in the same density as on normal non-PWS skin, in areas of skin previously occupied by PWS which was subsequently treated and cleared by the pulsed dye laser.

We postulate that the absence of varicella lesions in untreated or partially treated PWS could be related to the decrease or absence of nerves around PWS vessels,[12] preventing dissemination of the virus to the PWS skin. This might, in part, explain the appearance of varicella lesions in skin cleared of

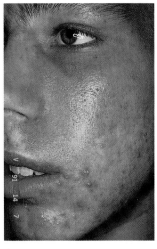

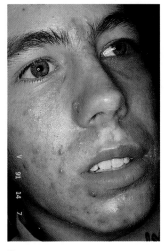

Fig. 6–13. *A.* The acne lesions extend as far as the margin of the PWS on the left side of the face. *B.* By contrast, acne lesions are present high up on the cheek on the non-PWS side of the face.

A   B

PWS following pulsed dye laser treatment. It has been demonstrated that the pulsed dye laser vascular injury induced at 577 or 585 nm is unique in that it selectively destroys the ectatic PWS vessels, replacing them with histologically "normal-appearing" vessels, presumably innervated by "normal" perivascular neurons.[13] The latter would provide a means for the virus to disseminate into the skin.

In summary, the pulsed dye laser has successfully treated adult patients with PWS. In contrast to other laser techniques, the pulsed dye laser treatments are multiple, and the progress is slow. Despite these perceived disadvantages, the skin treated by this laser is cleared of the PWS and retains its normal texture, color, markings, and elasticity.

References

1. Wilson AM, Kilpatrick R, Eckert H, et al. Thyroid neoplasms following irradiation. Br Med J 2:929, 1958.
2. Brauner G, Schliftman A, Cosman B. Evaluation of argon laser surgery in children under 13 years of age. Plast Reconstr Surg 87:37, 1991.
3. Alster TS, Kurban AK, Grove GL, Grove MJ, Tan OT. Alteration of argon laser induced PWS by the pulsed dye laser. Manuscript in preparation.
4. Noe JM, Barsky SH, Geer DE, et al. Portwine stains and the response to argon laser therapy: successful treatment of the predictive role of color, age and biopsy. Plast Reconstr Surg 65:130, 1980.
5. Dixon J, Huether S, Rotering RH. Hypertrophic scarring in argon laser treatment of portwine stains. Plast Reconstr Surg 73:771, 1984.
6. Tan OT, Sherwood K, Gilchrest BA. Treatment of children with portwine stains using the flashlamp-pumped dye laser. N Engl J Med 320:416, 1989.
7. Ashinoff R, Geronemus RG. Flashlamp-pumped pulsed dye laser for port wine stains in infancy: earlier versus later treatment. J Am Acad Dermatol 24:467, 1991.
8. Tan OT, Morrison P, Kurban AK. 585 nm for the treatment of port-wine stains. Plast Reconstr Surg 86:112, 1990.
9. Morelli JG, Tan OT, Garden JM, et al. Tunable dye laser (577 nm) treatment of portwine stains. Lasers Surg Med 6:94, 1986.
10. Tan OT, Stafford TJ. Treatment of port wine stains at 577 nm. Med Instrum 21:218, 1987.
11. Tang SV, Gilchrest BA, Noe JM, et al. In vivo spectrophotometric evaluation of normal, lesional and laser treated skin in patients with portwine stains. J Invest Dermatol 80:420, 1983.
12. Smoller BR, Rosen S. Port-wine stains: a disease of altered neural modulation of blood vessels. Arch Dermatol 122:177, 1986.
13. Tan OT, Whitaker D, Garden J, et al. Pulsed dye laser (577 nm) treatment of portwine stains: ultrastructural evidence of neovascularization and mast cell degranulation in healed lesions. J Invest Dermatol 90:395, 1988.

Chapter 7   Pulsed Dye Laser Treatment of Port-Wine Stains in Children

Joseph G. Morelli
William L. Weston

Earlier chapters in this text have discussed the pathophysiology of port-wine stains, nonpulsed dye laser treatments of port-wine stains, and the development of pulsed dye lasers for the treatment of these lesions. This chapter will concentrate on those aspects of port-wine stain (PWS) treatment using pulsed dye lasers which are important in the consideration of treatment of children.

Port-wine stains are congenital vascular malformations consisting of an increased number of ectatic capillaries within a given location of the skin. Their incidence is approximately 0.3%.[1] At birth, they usually present as light pink macules, although occasionally they will be dark red and elevated.[2] With time all PWS birthmarks mature by developing a deeper red color and progressive nodularity.[2] Along with the development of nodularity, port-wine stains can lead to hypertrophy of soft tissue and overgrowth of the affected area.[2] People afflicted with port-wine stains may suffer severe psychologic disturbances owing to the appearance of these malformations.[3] Thus, for both medical and psychologic reasons it has always been the goal to develop a method for eradication of these lesions at as early an age as possible.

The first goal of PWS laser therapy should be to begin treatment as soon as possible. Two recent reports contain evidence to support early treatment.[4,5] The first study demonstrated that children less than 7 years of age require fewer treatments to obtain clearing than do those children between the ages of 7 and 14 years.[4] The second study revealed that in patients less than 1 year of age, 83% of patients had greater than 50% clearing with 2.8 ± 1.4 treatments.[5] In the younger group there was no evidence for scarring, hypopigmentation, hyperpigmentation, or atrophy of the treated areas. From these studies, it is safe and more effective to begin treatments as early as possible. We prefer to begin treatments as early as 7 to 14 days of age. The optimal situation is one in which the child is first seen in consultation in the nursery. After discussion of the reasons for therapy and the benefit of early treatment, an appointment for the first treatment can be made within one week of discharge from the hospital.

More rapid clearing of the port-wine stain is only one reason for beginning treatments at as early an age as possible. Although port-wine stains do not enlarge beyond their original borders, they do grow with the child. Given a fixed laser beam diameter of 5 mm, the smaller the lesion, the fewer total laser pulses are required to treat the entire area.

Further, babies have no apprehension about the upcoming laser treatment. Babies are smaller and easier to handle, thereby allowing the entire PWS birthmark to be treated safely and quickly without the need for anesthesia. If treatments are begun within the first 2 weeks of life, then 3 treatments can be done before the child reaches 6 months of age. This should on the average clear 50% of the lesion. Three more treatments can then be done before one year of age. This would lead to marked improvement of all lesions before the child has been able to develop anxiety towards the treatment and the psychologic association that the port-wine stain is something abnormal.

The advantages of early treatment, then, are: (1) fewer treatments needed to clear the lesions; (2) fewer laser pulses required per individual treatment; (3) easy-to-perform treatment sessions without the need for anesthesia; (4) marked improvement by the age of 1 year.

Unfortunately, most children are not seen at an early age. We feel that this occurs for two main reasons. The first is the hesitancy of pediatricians and family practitioners to refer their patients for ''surgery'' at such a young age. This is likely related to the previous teaching that argon laser treatments were not effective in young children. The second reason is a lack of knowledge of the different types of vascular birthmarks. Many pediatric primary care givers counsel their patients that the vascular malformation will most likely resolve spontaneously. Although this may be true for the majority of hemangiomas, and the small salmon patches over the eyelids and forehead, it is definitely not true for the majority of macular pink/red port-wine stains noted in the newborn period. This is another reason why we feel it is important for parents to be urged to have a medical consultation during the time their child is in the newborn nursery; it would be helpful to clarify exactly which type of vascular lesion was present and to explain to the parents the natural history and treatment possibilities for the birthmark.

Given the facts that only a few patients with port-wine stain are seen within the first 6 months of life and that there is a large group of patients to whom the treatment was not available prior to 3 years ago, many patients between the ages of 6 months and 18 years present for treatment.

One of the debates concerning treatment of this group is whether general anesthesia should be used, and if so in what age groups it is indicated. Chapter 5 of this text details the options for anesthesia in laser surgery, so we will not discuss the types of anesthesia available. Although the majority of physicians performing laser surgery use some form of general anesthesia, especially on the 6-months to 12-year age group, we feel that it is not necessary for successful treatment; general anesthesia has never been used at our center. Because we do not use general anesthesia at our center, the remaining discussion will emphasize the approach to the laser treatment of port-wine stains in children without the use of general anesthesia.

Approach to the Treatment of Children

To be able to successfully treat children with port-wine stains using a pulsed dye laser, one must understand the developmental differences between the various age groups. The approach to treatment must be tailored to the age and personality of the individual patient. We prefer to begin by forming 5 broad categories. These are: (1) 0 to 18 months; (2) 18 months to 6 years; (3) 6 to 12 years; (4) greater than 12 years; (5) panic attack. We will start with the easiest group to deal with and move progressively to the more difficult challenges.

It is certainly easiest to treat the cooperative adolescent. A person in this age group is in the midst of difficult social adjustments. It is a time when any abnormality can be grossly overexaggerated. When an adolescent presents in consultation regarding treatment, he is usually ready to begin the therapy. During each treatment session, most of the lesion can be treated; this decreases the number of visits necessary to achieve clearing. One of the drawbacks in treating patients in this age group is that, because of school, they are less likely to come for treatments every 2 months. On the average they receive 3 or 4 treatments per year. Overall the treatment of these patients is simple and rewarding, although clearing will likely take 3 to 6 years.

The next easiest group to treat are the children between 2 weeks and 18 months of age. This is especially true for the subset of children less than 6 months of age. These patients lack apprehension when presenting for treatment. The child of this age cries during the treatment, but does not struggle very much. If the procedure has been properly explained to the parents, it can be performed quickly and efficiently. The patient immediately recovers following treatment, and the family can continue the day as if no procedure had been performed. The majority of the port-wine stain can be treated at every visit, and treatments can be performed every 2 months. Most of these patients will show greater than 50% lightening from 3 treatments.[5] Between the ages of 6 and 18 months the children progressively develop more anxiety toward the treatments. They also continue to increase in size and become more difficult to handle. As their total body size increases, so does the size of the port-wine stain, and thus more laser pulses are required to treat the lesion. Despite these facts it is still possible to treat a large area at each visit without much trouble.

The age groups 18 months to 6 years and 6 to 12 years are about equally difficult to treat, but for different reasons. As children reach 18 months of age, they clearly remember situations, surroundings, and faces. They often have a great deal of anxiety regarding the laser treatments. It is not unusual for them to begin crying at the sight of the clinic, the laser treatment room, or the physician. With this group the physician-patient interaction is very important. Although the children are old enough to understand the pain associated with the treatment, they are not old enough to understand an explanation of why the treatment is being performed. It is generally unrewarding, immediately before a treatment, to attempt to discuss with a patient in this age group the reasons that the treatments are being performed. The most efficient way to treat this group of patients is for everyone involved to have an understanding that the best results are achieved by performing the treatment as rapidly as possible. Once the treatment session has ended and the infliction of pain has ceased, it is time for the physician to spend time with the patient. It is helpful at this juncture to discuss how the child feels about the treatment and for the physician to show the child that he understands that the treatment is painful. It is also very important to attempt to have the child understand that the physician cares for the child, and that it is the laser treatment, not the physician, that is hurting the child. Despite this approach, the treatment sessions are still very traumatic. Most children accept this fact without too much difficulty and are only upset at the times immediately surrounding a scheduled appointment. Between appointments, they show no signs that going through the treatment has affected their lives. There is a small subset of this group for whom, everyone agrees, this approach to treatment is far too traumatic. The choices then become using general anesthesia or delaying treatments. As we have stated earlier, we are opposed to the use of general anesthesia for pulsed dye laser treatments. We also feel that the true advantage of early treatment is gained only when treatments are begun before 18 months of age, and that there is minimal gain regarding treatment efficacy whether the child is being treated at 4 or 7 years of age. Despite all the trauma associated with treating this subset of patients, many of their parents are anxious to finish the treatments as soon as possible. This is when all the options for treatment and the risks versus advantages must carefully be considered.

The children of grade school age are also very difficult to treat. Although they do understand why the treatments are being performed and usually really desire the removal of their birthmark, they tend to spend much more time between treatments thinking about the pain associated with the treatment and thus have a much greater anxiety level. They also have a greater need to feel in control of the situation. Unlike the previous group, it is more rewarding to spend time with these children before beginning the treatment sessions. Options for treatment can be discussed, such as: how many total pulses will be done during this session; what area will be treated; how many pulses will be done before taking a break; and how long each rest will be. Treatment sessions with this group of children can be painstakingly slow. Although it is important to give the child options regarding treatment, some children will attempt to bargain on even the smallest issue. Thus, it becomes equally important for the parents to have established firm guidelines for the physician to work within. Again, this approach will work with most of the children, but a few will be impossible to treat. For this age group we feel that if the child does not think that the treatments are worthwhile, then they should be delayed until the child truly desires the removal of the birthmark.

The last group is by far the most difficult to treat. ''Panic-attack'' patients usually are between the ages of 10 and 14 years. When they present for their initial treatment, they appear calm and collected and fully desire removal of the port-wine stain. The minute that the first treatment is about to begin, however, they become totally irrational and refuse to allow even one pulse to be done. Once this panic attack has begun it is nearly impossible to break. The parents should be told that this is an infrequent, yet unpredictable, response, and that it means that at this time the child is really not ready to begin the treatments.

University of Colorado Experience

Over the last 3 years we have treated 187 patients with port-wine stains under the age of 18 years. A total of 217,269 pulses have been done in 1,324 treatments. The overall average is 7 treatments per patient and 164 pulses per

Table 7–1. Pulsed Dye Laser Treatment of 187 PWS Patients Under 18 Years of Age

Patient age at beginning of treatment	Number of patients	Average number of treatments per patient	Average number of pulses per treatment
0–18 months	48	7.8	225
18 months–6 years	59	8.3	128
6–12 years	44	6.2	123
>12 years	36	5.3	197
Total	187	7.0	164

treatment (Table 7–1). The most treatments per patient were performed on the preschool children, and the most pulses per treatment on the children less than 18 months and those greater than 12 years old (Table 7–1).

Of all 187 patients, 55 either have transferred or have not returned for a visit for over 1 year and are unavailable for evaluation. A large proportion of these patients were those who came from an area which initially did not offer the laser treatment, but which since have acquired the laser. Of the remaining 132 patients, 17 (or 13%) have had complete removal of their port-wine stains. Dividing the patients by age reveals that it is optimal to begin treatment as early as possible. In those patients that began treatment before they were 18 months of age, 25% have had total PWS clearing as compared to 7–10% for the other groups (Table 7–2).

The success of early treatment is likely to result from various factors. As has previously been shown, those children treated at an earlier age require fewer retreatments.[4,5] Also, patients of this age group do not attend school and can come for treatments frequently. Further, it is easier to do larger treatment areas at each visit, and because the children are smaller, this frequently covers the entire port-wine stain (Table 7–2).

Among the children over the age of 6 whose port-wine stain is totally resolved, 3 of the 4 had central forehead lesions. They all resolved with 3 or fewer treatments. In general, these port-wine stains tend to be smaller and lighter than many of those located in other areas (Fig. 7–1).

Table 7–2. Total PWS Clearing With Pulsed Dye Laser Treatment by Age Group

Age at beginning Rx	Number of patients	Percentage PWS completely eliminated
0–18 months	36	25
18 months–6 years	40	10
6–12 years	30	7
>12 years	28	7
Total	134	13

Fig. 7–1. *A,C,E.* Port-wine stains prior to laser treatments. *B,D,F.* Post dye laser treatments. Note that the treated skin is indistinguishable from adjacent normal skin.

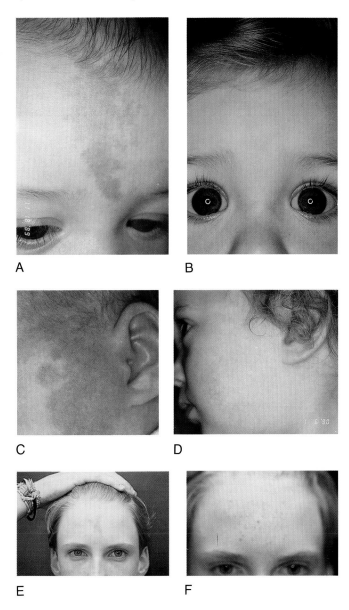

Conclusion

Port-wine stains in children are now easily treatable. There is mounting evidence that the optimal results are obtained if one begins treatments as early in life as possible (Fig. 7–1). We have performed the initial treatment on children as young as 1 week of life.

We recommend that all children with vascular malformations be evaluated in the nursery. This will accomplish many goals. Port-wine stains can be differentiated from hemangiomas or other vascular malformations. If a child has a facial port-wine stain, the parents can be counseled on the risks of ophthalmologic or central nervous system complications.[6] Details of the PWS laser treatment and the importance of early treatment can be discussed.

References

1. Jacobs AH, Walton RG. The incidence of birthmarks in the neonate. Pediatrics 58:218, 1976.
2. Geronemus RG, Ashinoff R. The medical necessity of evaluation and treatment of port wine stains. J Dermatol Surg Onc 17:76, 1991.
3. Heller A, Rafmans S, Zvagulis I, Pless IB. Birth defects and psychosocial adjustments. Am J Dis Child 139:257, 1985.
4. Tan OT, Sherwood K, Gilchrest BA. Treatment of children with port-wine stains using the flashlamp-pumped tunable dye laser. N Engl J Med 320:416, 1989.
5. Ashinoff R, Geronemus RG. Flashlamp-pumped pulsed dye laser for port wine stains in infancy: earlier versus later treatment. J Am Acad Dermatol 24:467, 1991.
6. Talman B, Tan OT, Morelli JG, et al. Location of port-wine stains and the likelihood of ophthalmic and/or central nervous system complications. Pediatrics 87:323, 1991.

Chapter 8   Ophthalmologic Monitoring of Port-Wine Stain and Hemangioma Patients

Douglas R. Fredrick
Lois E.H. Smith

Cutaneous vascular lesions involving the periocular region pose special diagnostic and therapeutic challenges. Two of the most common types of lesions are the port-wine stain of Sturge-Weber syndrome and juvenile hemangiomas. These two vascular malformations have different clinical features; both are associated with different forms of ocular disorder. The port-wine stain is associated with glaucoma. The periocular juvenile hemangiomas can cause distortion of the shape of the globe and/or occlusion of the visual axis, which can severely affect visual development. Thus, early detection and management of both lesions are crucial. When present, these ocular manifestations occur in early infancy and childhood, and thus the patients rarely complain of ocular or visual symptoms. For this reason, close surveillance of patients with periocular vascular malformations by an ophthalmologist from the onset of detection is mandatory to prevent and treat these vision-threatening conditions.

Nevus Flammeus of Sturge-Weber Syndrome

Sturge-Weber syndrome, also designated as "encephalotrigeminal angiomatosis" and "angio-encephalo-cutaneous syndrome," describes the syndrome of facial angioma with ipsilateral intracranial hemangioma. Facial involvement (and eye involvement) can occur without intracranial involvement. A significant percentage of these patients have associated ocular pathologic symptoms, and of those with ocular involvement glaucoma occurs in 30% of patients.[1] The pathologic findings of facial and intracranial angioma have been described earlier, and the specific ocular findings will be discussed more completely in this chapter.

All parts of the eye and visual system can be affected in Sturge-Weber syndrome; glaucoma, however, is the most common finding. Schirmer in 1860 was the first to describe a patient with facial angioma and buphthalmos (ox-eye). Buphthalmos is generalized enlargement of the eye that occurs as a result of congenital glaucoma with increased intraocular pressure. In surveys of patients with Sturge-Weber syndrome the incidence of glaucoma is found to be 30 to 40%. If the facial angioma involves the lids and ocular adnexa, the risk for development of glaucoma is higher compared to patients without periocular involvement. Anderson's rule states that if the upper lid is involved the risk of intraocular involvement is much higher than if the upper lid is spared.[2] Engorgement of episcleral and conjunctival vessels, however, can often be difficult to evaluate; thus all patients with facial nevus flammeus should initially be considered equally at risk for development of glaucoma and subject to close surveillance.

It is important to note that glaucoma can manifest itself in different ways in patients with facial nevus flammeus. Classically, the glaucoma presents as buphthalmos—a grossly enlarged eye present soon after birth owing to increased intraocular pressure. Historically, this has been the mode of presentation in 70 to 80% of the patients with glaucoma associated with Sturge-Weber syndrome. In the other 20 to 30% of the cases, increased intraocular pressure without gross enlargement of the eye may occur. Glaucoma can develop later in infancy and up through childhood and adolescence. A recent survey found that glaucoma developed after the age of 4 years in 44% of all cases.[3] This indicates that the absence of glaucoma early in life does not preclude its development later in life, so these patients must have long-term surveillance with frequent measurement of intraocular pressure.

The causal mechanism of glaucoma in patients with Sturge-Weber syndrome is not clearly understood. There are two theories which attempt to explain the glaucoma, and each theory has been supported by clinical experience and pathologic findings. These theories will be better understood after a brief explanation of ocular fluid dynamics and homeostasis. Normal intraocular pressure is maintained by the eye's constant production and filtering of aqueous humor. Aqueous humor, produced by the ciliary body, flows forward around the lens through the pupil and is filtered out through the trabecular meshwork. After passing through the trabecular meshwork it enters Schlemm's canal, which connects to the venous system via collector channels. The rate of aqueous-humor production is regulated on a diurnal curve that is usually fairly constant but can vary markedly in patients with choroidal hemangiomas. The rate of filtration depends on the resistance to outflow through the trabecular tissues and the pressure gradient from the intraocular pressure into the episcleral venous pressure.

The first theory proposes that glaucoma in Sturge-Weber syndrome is a variant of congenital glaucoma and is a result of abnormal structure of the trabecular meshwork. During clinical examinations aberrant stromal material overlying the trabecular meshwork has been described.[4] Pathologic specimens taken from buphthalmic eyes have documented anomalous trabecular meshwork tissue as well as premature aging changes in the tissue.[5] These findings are more often found in patients who present with buphthalmos and glaucoma early in life. Some patients, however, have normal gonioscopic findings and normal pathologic findings on examination of meshwork specimens, suggesting an alternate mechanism is at work.

The second proposed mechanism of glaucoma stems from the finding that episcleral venous pressure is elevated in patients with Sturge-Weber syndrome. Often it is easy to visualize the engorged episcleral and conjunctival vessels on the surface of the eye. When measurement of episcleral pressure has been performed on these patients, the values have been found elevated compared to contralateral or uninvolved eyes.[6] This can lead to increased resistance of outflow and thus increased intraocular pressure. Most likely the cause for glaucoma is multifactorial, with both of the above mechanisms involved.

Glaucoma left untreated in children can lead to optic nerve damage, corneal edema, significant refractive error, ocular enlargement, and, finally, irreversible vision loss. With the awareness of the high incidence of glaucoma in patients with Sturge-Weber syndrome, pediatricians should refer these patients to an ophthalmologist for evaluation as soon as the diagnosis is made. A complete ophthalmic examination should be performed, with special attention paid to intraocular pressure, gonioscopic findings, corneal diameter, and optic nerve appearance. It may be necessary to examine children under anesthesia in order to facilitate a complete examination. If no glaucoma is detected, the patient should be re-examined every 3 to 4 months. If glaucoma is detected, treatment should be instituted immediately.

The management of glaucoma in patients with Sturge-Weber syndrome is difficult, as the glaucoma often proves refractory to conventional treatment. The first line of therapy is medical management, including topical and oral medications. Many of the patients will not be controlled with medical therapy and will require surgical intervention to lower the pressure. The success of such procedures is limited in this population, and many patients require numerous surgical procedures.[3,7] Because these patients often have coexistent periocular and choroidal hemangiomas, there is a higher complication rate in performing intraocular surgery on patients with Sturge-Weber syndrome. It is important that ophthalmologists managing these patients be prepared to handle the complications. Some of the surgical procedures utilized to control pressure are: goniotomy and trabeculotomy — cutting open trabecular tissues to facilitate outflow of aqueous humor; trabeculectomy — creating a surgical fistula to allow fluid to drain out of the eye into surrounding ocular tissues; and implanting filtering setons — synthetic valves which conduct fluid out of the eye into surrounding tissues. It is sometimes necessary to decrease aqueous production by treating the ciliary body with cryotherapy. Fifteen to thirty per cent of Sturge-Weber syndrome patients with glaucoma will have severe visual impairment despite maximal therapy; but with early detection, close surveillance, and timely intervention many patients with glaucoma can maintain excellent vision.

The ocular findings of Sturge-Weber syndrome are not limited to glaucoma and can involve all parts of the eye. The angioma of the lids can become nodular with age and create ptosis. The conjunctival and episcleral vessels may be tortuous and dilated. The iris of the involved eye may be more deeply pigmented, and iris colobomas and anisocoria have been described.[8] A common finding, described in 40% of patients with Sturge-Weber syndrome, is the presence of choroidal hemangioma. Choroidal hemangiomas create a characteristic red appearance in the fundus described as a ''tomato catsup'' fundus.[9] Hemangiomas of the choroid are associated with exudation of fluid and sensory retinal detachments, which can lead to permanent visual loss. Treatment includes use of laser therapy, periocular steroids, and, rarely, external beam radiation.[10] Finally, the intracranial angioma often involves the occipital cortex and can lead to progressive calcification. The cerebral atrophy that follows can leave the patient with homonymous hemianopias.

In summary it can be said that Sturge-Weber syndrome can affect or harm the eye and vision in many different ways. The presentation of ocular manifestations with Sturge-Weber syndrome is varied as is the natural history of the disease. Close ophthalmologic surveillance of these patients with early detection and treatment of ocular disease can help prevent permanent ocular damage and visual loss.

Capillary Hemangiomas of Eyelid

Capillary hemangiomas are the most common form of hemangioma, occurring in 1 of every 200 live births. They are the most common adnexal vascular tumor of childhood, more common in females than males. The lesions are usually superficial and elevated, and they exhibit a reddish-purple color with soft consistency. Deeper lesions may have a blue coloration or no discoloration at all. Histologically, these tumors are composed of lobules of capillaries of plump endothelial cells that tend to obliterate the vascular lumina.[10a] The natural history of these lesions on the lid is similar to that of such lesions located elsewhere; that is, they usually appear in the first 2 months of life and enlarge rapidly in the first 6 months of life. Spontaneous regression occurs over the ensuing several years. The lesions are more often found on the upper lid, occurring there 60% of the time, but can occur anywhere in the ocular adnexa.[11] Whereas most capillary hemangiomas of the skin are only a cosmetic problem, hemangiomas involving the eyelids and orbit can cause severe and permanent visual impairment if not recognized and treated. The most important and feared complication of periocular hemangioma is the induction of amblyopia. Amblyopia—"dullness of vision"—is defined as a unilateral or bilateral decrease of visual acuity caused by form vision deprivation and/or abnormal binocular interactions for which no organic causes can be determined by the physical examination of the eye and which in appropriate cases is reversible by therapeutic measures.[11a] There are three mechanisms for the development of amblyopia, and capillary hemangioma can cause amblyopia in each.

The most obvious way in which hemangiomas cause amblyopia is by occluding the visual axis by blocking the pupil. This leads to amblyopia ex anopsia, or visual deprivation amblyopia. At birth the visual pathways and visual cortex are immature and not fully developed. Development occurs for the first several years of life, and focused retinal images are required to have normal cortical development. If the image is occluded during this sensitive period, the visual cortex will not develop properly, and amblyopia will ensue. The earlier in life the occlusion, and the greater the duration of occlusion, the more profound the amblyopia and the more difficult it is to reverse the amblyopia with patching therapy. If more than several weeks of occlusion occur in the first few months of life, severe visual loss can result. Thus, it is not surprising to see that, in surveys of patients with lid hemangiomas, those with the worst visual acuity are those who had complete occlusion for the longest duration.[12] Moreover, those patients with the worst visual acuity generally had inadequate treatment of amblyopia—patching therapy that was initiated too late and not compliantly performed. If the hemangioma is causing occlusion of the visual axis, treatment of the lesion must be initiated and patching therapy begun as soon as the occlusion is removed. Weeks of delay can be crucial.

The second mechanism by which amblyopia may develop is by having unequal refractive errors between the two eyes—''anisometropic amblyopia.'' Robb was the first to demonstrate that asymmetry of refractive error is common, occurring in 46% of all hemangioma patients surveyed.[13] Patients with lid hemangiomas tend to be more myopic and have greater amounts of astigmatism in the involved eye. Astigmatism, i.e., irregular corneal curvature, results from the physical pressure of the hemangioma on the cornea. Amblyopia develops in a large percentage of these eyes, but fortunately it can be treated with spectacle therapy and patching therapy. It has also been shown that astigmatism may decrease if the hemangiomas are treated early and respond to treatment.

The third causal mechanism of amblyopia results from unequal ocular alignment, giving rise to strabismic amblyopia. Strabismus is seen in 30 to 40% of patients with lid hemangiomas referred to tertiary centers. Many of these patients had hemangiomas involving the orbit with direct involvement with the extraocular muscles. Here again, patching therapy, treatment of angioma, and surgical straightening of the eyes can help restore vision in these amblyopic eyes.

It is important to realize that although treatment of amblyopia is often successful in restoring vision, prevention of amblyopia is the larger goal. When a child presents with a hemangioma involving either the upper or the lower eyelid, he should be referred to an *ophthalmologist* promptly even if there appears to be no occlusion of the visual axis. Refractive errors can be detected only by performing a dilated, complete ophthalmic exam. If anisometropia, astigmatism, or strabismus is detected, therapy will be directed at treating the lesion, and patching therapy may be instituted to prevent amblyopia from developing. If no ocular problems are found, the child should be re-examined frequently to detect growth of the lesion and possible development of ocular disorder.

The treatment of capillary hemangiomas has improved greatly in the past decade. Prior to 1980, therapeutic interventions were often unsuccessful, morbid procedures. Surgical debulking would often result in poorly functioning eyelids and cosmetically disfiguring scars. Intralesional injection of sclerosing agents often led to necrosis of tissue and recurrence of lesion as well as severe pain. External beam radiotherapy was often successful at causing shrinkage of the hemangioma, but side effects of radiation on the eye, including dry eye, possible cataract formation, atrophy of skin, and potential nerve and retinal damage, were always worrisome. In the 1970s, the use of systemic corticosteroids was found to hasten the regression of capillary hemangiomas.[14,15] Even though this was found to be an effective therapy, recurrence of the hemangioma after cessation of treatment was not uncommon, placing children at risk for the systemic side effects of corticosteroid therapy.

In the 1980s, the use of intralesional corticosteroid injection for capillary hemangiomas was first described. Subsequent study has shown that this is a safe and effective mode of therapy that leads to rapid regression of tumor in a majority of cases.[16,17] Triamcinolone is injected directly into the lesion using a 30-gauge needle. This can be done with the patient awake and restrained or under masked inhalational anesthesia. Frequently there is initial swelling of the lesion, but regression begins rapidly, usually within 1 week of injection. A second treatment is sometimes necessary if the lesion fails to regress the desired amount. Rarely are more than two treatment sessions required. Clinically effective steroids are the angiostatic steroids hydrocortisone and triamcinolone.

The mechanism by which steroids induce regression of these vascular tumors is not known. Some have speculated that steroids may induce arterial or capillary constriction in addition to affecting endothelial cells directly and inhibiting the growth of blood vessels.[18] Regardless of the mechanism, this has been found to be a safe and efficacious procedure. The use of short-acting, locally deposited corticosteroid lessens the risk of systemic side effects of long-term systemic corticosteroid therapy. Complications are uncommon, but some have been reported. There has been one case of eyelid necrosis following local steroid injection,[19] and there has been one reported case of central retinal artery occlusion following injection of periocular corticosteroid.[20] In order to minimize the risk of this complication, it has been recommended to inject the steroids slowly in multiple 0.1 ml aliquots and to avoid firm digital pressure on the lesion. Complications are rare, and intralesional steroid therapy remains the treatment of choice for periocular capillary hemangiomas. A new mode of therapy is currently under investigation for the treatment of hemangiomas unresponsive to corticosteroids. Alpha interferon has been shown to lead to tumor regression in a large level of variety tumors. This therapy, still in the research stage, holds promise for the treatment of hemangiomas resistant to conventional therapy.

Hemangiomas involving the eyelids can sometimes be more extensive than they appear, extending into the orbit. Orbital hemangiomas may cause proptosis with secondary exposure keratopathy, compression of the optic nerve, and infiltration of extraocular muscles with strabismus. Diagnostically, orbital hemangioma poses a challenging problem; conditions included in the differential diagnosis are lymphangioma, neurofibromatosis, and rhabdomyosarcoma.[21,11] Computed axial tomography and magnetic resonance imaging help in the diagnosis. Biopsies should be performed if the clinical diagnosis is not certain. Orbital hemangiomas should not be treated by direct intralesional injection for fear of inducing a retrobulbar hemorrhage. These lesions may require treatment by systemic steroids or surgical excision.

Summary

Cutaneous vascular lesions involving the eyelid can be associated with and cause serious ocular disease. Patients with facial port-wine stains— commonly referred to as Sturge-Weber syndrome—should be seen by an ophthalmologist as soon as the diagnosis is made. They will require long-term ophthalmic monitoring to detect and treat glaucoma, which occurs in a large percentage of these patients. Treatment of glaucoma can be difficult, requiring constant vigilance on the part of the ophthalmologist. Patients with capillary hemangioma involving the eyelid should be seen by an ophthalmologist promptly. Treatment of the lesion should be instituted to prevent, or treat, amblyopia. Patching and spectacle therapy for amblyopia is as important as the treatment of the vascular lesion if vision is to be restored and preserved. The ophthalmologist should join the dermatologist and pediatrician in a multidisciplinary approach to the treatment of vascular lesions involving the eyelid.

References

1. Duke-Elder S. System of Ophthalmology Vol XI. St Louis, Mosby, 1969, pp 637–645.
2. Anderson JR. Hydrophthalmia or Congenital Glaucoma: Its Causes, Treatment and Outlook. Cambridge, Mass Univ Press, 1939, pp 180–221.
3. Iwach AG, et al. Analysis of surgical and medical management of glaucoma in Sturge-Weber syndrome. Ophthalmology 97:904, 1990.
4. Barkan O. Goniotomy for glaucoma associated with nevus flammeus. Am J Ophthalmol 43:545, 1957.
5. Cibis GW, Tripathi RA, Tripathi BJ. Glaucoma in Sturge-Weber syndrome. Ophthalmology 91:1061, 1984.
6. Phelps CD. The pathogenesis of glaucoma in Sturge-Weber syndrome. Ophthalmology 85:276, 1978.
7. Walton DS. Hemangioma of the Lid. *In* Glaucoma. Edited by P.A. Chandler. Philadelphia, Lea & Febiger, 1979.
8. Font RL, Ferry AP. Phakomatosis. Int Ophthalmol Clin Vol 12, 1972.
9. Susac JO, et al. The "tomato catsup" fundus in Sturge-Weber syndrome. Arch Ophthalmol 92:69, 1974.
10. Plowman PN, Harnett AN. The radiotherapy in benign orbital disease. I: complicated ocular angiomas. Br J Ophthalmol 72:286, 1988.
10a. Spencer WH, ed. Ophthalmic Pathology: An Atlas and Textbook. 3rd ed. Philadelphia, WB Saunders, 1985.
11. Haik BG, et al. Capillary hemangioma of the lids and orbit: an analysis of the clinical features and therapeutic results in 101 cases. Ophthalmology 86:760, 1979.
11a. Van Noorder GK. Binocular Vision and Ocular Motility. St. Louis, Mosby, 1990, 208.
12. Stigmar EG, et al. Ophthalmic sequelae of infantile hemangiomas of the eyelids and orbit. Am J Ophthalmol 85:806, 1978.
13. Robb RN. Refractive errors associated with hemangioma of the eyelids and orbit in infancy. Am J Ophthalmol 83:52, 1977.
14. de Venecia G, Lobeck CC. Successful treatment of eyelid hemangioma with prednisone. Arch Ophthalmol 84:98, 1970.
15. Hiles DA, Pilchard WA. Corticosteroid control of neonatal hemangiomas of the orbit and ocular adnexa. Am J Ophthalmol 1971:1003, 1971.
16. Kushner BJ. Intralesional corticosteroid injection for infantile adnexal hemangioma. Am J Ophthalmol 93:496, 1982.
17. Zak TA, and Morin JD. Early local steroid therapy of infantile eyelid hemangiomas. J Pediatr Ophthalmol Strabismus 18:25, 1971.
18. Folkman J. Successful treatment of an angiogenic disease. N Engl J Med 320:1211, 1989.
19. Sutula FC, Glover AT. Eyelid necrosis following intralesional corticosteroid injection for capillary hemangioma. Ophthalmic Surg 18:103, 1987.
20. Shorr N, Seiff SR. Central retinal artery occlusion associated with periocular corticosteroid injection for juvenile hemangioma. Ophthalmic Surg 17:229, 1986.
21. Iliff WJ. Orbital lymphangiomas. Ophthalmology 86:914, 1979.

Chapter 9 Neurologic Manifestations of Sturge-Weber Syndrome

E. Steven Roach

Only about one fourth of patients with facial port-wine nevi have neurologic dysfunction resulting from leptomeningeal and vascular brain lesions.[1] The combination of an intracranial lesion and the facial cutaneous angioma constitutes *Sturge-Weber syndrome*. Specific signs and symptoms vary considerably from patient to patient, but classically include epileptic seizures, mental retardation, and hemiparesis.[2,3] Sturge-Weber syndrome occurs sporadically—there are no well-described examples of the complete syndrome in more than one member of a family.

It is generally accepted that only patients whose facial angioma includes the upper face have a substantial risk for neurologic impairment, while intracranial lesions are almost never found with cutaneous angiomas limited to the face below the lower eyelid.[4,5] However, several patients with an intracranial angioma but without cutaneous involvement have been described.[5-8] Other patients with refractory epilepsy and occipital calcifications, but no cutaneous nevus, probably have this same syndrome.[9] The brain lesion is usually found ipsilateral to the facial nevus, although there are occasional exceptions. Bilateral brain lesions are found in 15% of patients, including some with unilateral cutaneous nevi.[10] Although the extent of the cutaneous lesion correlates poorly with the severity of neurologic disease,[5] there is some evidence that children with a bilateral nevus have a greater likelihood of neurologic involvement[4] and tend to have an earlier onset of seizures.[11] Despite earlier assertions, any link between the facial nevus and the sensory distribution of the trigeminal nerve is coincidental.

Neurologic Manifestations

Most patients with Sturge-Weber syndrome are neurologically normal for several months or even years,[12] although occasional newborns have neurologic difficulty.[13,14] Typically, epileptic seizures and hemiparesis develop acutely during the first two or three years of life, often in conjunction with a febrile illness. Focal motor seizures or generalized tonic-clonic seizures are most typical of Sturge-Weber syndrome initially, but infantile spasms, myoclonic seizures, and atonic seizures sometimes occur.[15-17] In older children and adults, complex partial seizures and focal motor seizures predominate.

Epileptic seizures occur in 72% of Sturge-Weber patients with unilateral lesions and in 93% of patients with bihemispheric involvement.[11] Although seizures from Sturge-Weber syndrome may be difficult to fully control with anticonvulsant medications, the clinical severity is highly variable. Some patients continue to have daily seizures after the initial deterioration in spite of various daily anticonvulsant medications. Others have long seizure-free intervals, sometimes even without medication, punctuated by periods of status epilepticus or clusters of intense seizure activity.[17] Some patients' seizures can be controlled with the newer anticonvulsant medications, particularly with careful attention to dosing schedules and serum drug levels. Generally patients with severe neurologic impairment tend to have more refractory epileptic seizures than those with normal intelligence and no focal neurologic deficits. The converse is also true: patients without seizures are seldom if ever mentally retarded. Onset of seizures prior to 2 years of age tends to increase the likelihood of future mental retardation and refractory epilepsy, but exceptions to this rule are common.

Mental deficiency occurs in about half of Sturge-Weber patients,[5,18,19] although with bilateral brain involvement only 8% are normal.[11] The degree of intellectual impairment ranges from mild to profound; behavioral abnormalities are sometimes a problem even in patients who are not mentally retarded. In general, patients with refractory seizures are much more likely to be mentally retarded, and patients who have never had seizures are typically normal. There is little doubt that uncontrolled epileptic seizures account for at least a portion of the intellectual impairment in these children. However, the extent and location of the vascular lesion in the brain is also important: an extensive lesion may well promote more difficult seizures *and* intellectual impairment. In favor of this argument is the increased likelihood of seizures and retardation in patients with bilateral lesions.[11]

Hemiparesis often develops in conjunction with the initial flurry of seizure activity. Although usually attributed to postictal weakness, the hemiparesis often persists much longer than the few hours typical of a postictal deficit and may remain as permanent hemiparesis. Other patients suddenly develop weakness without seizures, either as repeated episodes of weakness similar to transient ischemic attacks or as a single strokelike episode with persistent deficit.[20] Children who develop hemiparesis early in life usually have arrested growth in the weak extremities.

Other focal neurologic deficits depend on the anatomic site and extent of the intracranial vascular lesion. Because the occipital region is frequently involved, visual field deficits are a particular problem.[19] Patients with glaucoma are doubly at risk, because they may become amblyopic in one or both eyes from the glaucoma and have superimposed visual field loss from the brain lesion.

Hydrocephalus is a rare complication of Sturge-Weber syndrome.[13,21] Fishman and Baram described one child who initially had macrocephaly without ventriculomegaly but later developed hydrocephalus.[22] The cerebral angiogram demonstrated dilated superficial cortical veins but nonfilling of the deep venous channels ipsilateral to the angioma. Impaired venous drainage is the likely mechanism of progressive macrocephaly in these children.[22,23]

Intracranial hemorrhage is not a significant problem in Sturge-Weber patients. Anderson and Duncan presented one adult with subarachnoid hemorrhage probably caused by Sturge-Weber syndrome.[24] Microscopic hemorrhages are mentioned in autopsy series but probably have limited clinical significance. In 1906, Cushing described three patients that he assumed had spontaneous hemorrhage, but all three developed sudden seizures and weakness fairly typical of the pattern now seen during the initial neurologic deterioration in children without hemorrhage. Even with operative or postmortem examination of the brain in two of these patients, no direct evidence of hemorrhage was found. Cushing, incidentally, ligated the external carotid artery of one patient as a preliminary to brain surgery and noted that the nevus blanched immediately, remaining so for 48 hours before regaining its red color.[25]

The mechanism of neurologic deterioration in Sturge-Weber patients is still debated. Chronic hypoxia of the cerebral cortex adjacent to the angioma resulting from reduced blood flow has been postulated. Increased metabolic requirements during seizures could potentiate the oxygen deficit.[19] Frequent epileptic seizures per se no doubt contribute to impaired neurologic function in some children, for this phenomenon is also noted in children with refractory seizures from a variety of underlying causes. Neurologic impairment usually lasts too long to be a transient postictal deficit. Repeated venous occlusions may account for the saltatory deterioration suffered by some patients as well as transient neurologic dysfunction.[20] Venous thrombosis could also explain the typical first episode of neurologic dysfunction: venous occlusion from any cause often produces epileptic seizures together with a focal neurologic deficit that often slowly resolves, much like the initial episode of dysfunction in Sturge-Weber patients.[3] It is likely that all these factors may play some role, singly or in combination, in neurologic deterioration in Sturge-Weber patients.

Diagnostic Evaluation

Since only a few children with facial port-wine nevi have an intracranial angioma, neuroimaging studies and other tests help to distinguish these children with Sturge-Weber syndrome from those with an isolated cutaneous lesion.[2] This distinction is all-important for establishing an accurate diagnosis and prognosis, and for this reason thorough testing is probably justifiable during the initial evaluation. Neuroimaging, electroencephalography, and functional testing with positron emission tomography (PET) and single photon emission computed tomography (SPECT) may also help to define the extent of the intracranial lesion for possible epilepsy surgery.[26,27]

The radiographic finding most suggestive of Sturge-Weber syndrome is gyriform calcification adjacent to the leptomeningeal angioma. Extensive calcification can be visualized with plain radiographs,[28] but computed cranial tomography is a far more sensitive means of identifying calcification.[7,16,29] The leptomeningeal lesion is more likely to occur posteriorly, although

Fig. 9–1. Computed cranial tomography from patient with left facial port-wine nevus and ipsilateral leptomeningeal lesion. Note the gyriform pattern of the calcification in the left posterior hemisphere. (Reproduced from Garcia et al.,[20] with permission.)

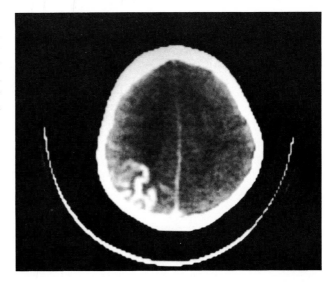

anterior lesions or extensive abnormalities of the entire hemisphere are relatively common (Fig. 9–1). Contrast enhancement of the brain adjacent to the calcification and enlargement of the deep vascular channels are sometimes noted.[30] Ipsilateral enlargement of the choroid plexus is an occasional feature of Sturge-Weber syndrome. Cerebral atrophy is apparent with computed tomography especially if the atrophy is extensive or progressive.

Subtle atrophy is more readily demonstrated by magnetic resonance imaging, which demonstrates cerebral calcifications poorly if at all. Recent reports suggest that magnetic resonance imaging with gadolinium contrast (Fig. 9–2) provides a subtle indicator of the abnormal intracranial vessels in Sturge-Weber patients.[31–33] This observation could prove quite significant if it allows the diagnosis to be made early with a safe noninvasive test. The use of magnetic resonance angiography to directly image the larger abnormal vessels is an intriguing but as yet untested possibility.

Cerebral arteriography is no longer routinely required for the evaluation of Sturge-Weber syndrome, but it may be of use in atypical patients or prior to surgery for epilepsy. Occasional patients have evidence of arterial occlusion,[34–36] and one patient may have had an arteriovenous malformation.[37] The arterial phase of angiography, however, is typically normal.[38] The venous abnormalities are more obvious. The superficial cortical veins are reduced in number (Fig. 9–3) and the deep draining veins are often dilated and tortuous. Failure of the sagittal sinus to opacify after ipsilateral carotid injection may be secondary to obliteration of the superficial cortical veins,[39] and the abnormal deep venous channels probably have a similar origin as they form collateral conduits for nonfunctioning cortical veins.[38,39] Similar deep venous collaterals have been described after thrombosis of the sagittal sinus and cortical veins.[40] Bentson and colleagues believe that the lack of functioning cortical veins in Sturge-Weber patients is probably the result of thrombosis.[39]

Electroencephalography (EEG) typically reveals depressed amplitude of electrical activity adjacent to the leptomeningeal angioma.[15,41] Focal epileptic discharges may be recorded either ipsilateral[41] or contralateral[15] to the

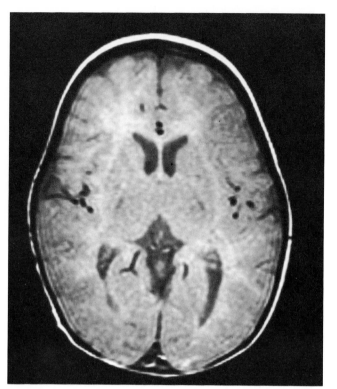

A

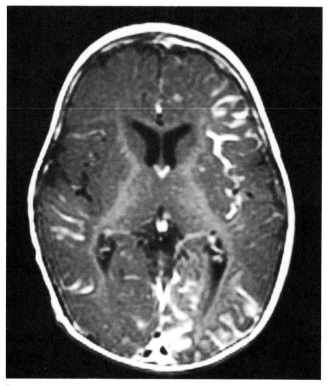

B

Fig. 9–2. A. The cranial magnetic resonance scan from a patient with Sturge-Weber syndrome is normal at the level of the anterior horns of the lateral ventricles. B. The addition of gadolinium contrast in this same patient reveals the left leptomeningeal lesion and extensive intraparenchymal vascular abnormalities. (Reproduced from Roach,[55] with permission.)

Fig. 9–3. In the venous phase of the left carotid angiogram of a patient with Sturge-Weber syndrome there are no cortical veins in left occipital region. The arterial phase was normal. (Reproduced from Garcia et al.,[20] with permission.)

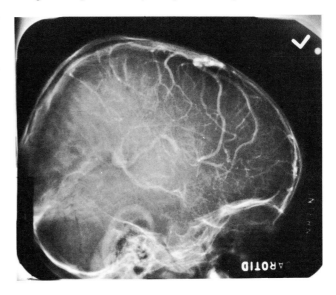

affected hemisphere. Synchronous bilateral EEG discharges are sometimes recorded even in patients with involvement of only one hemisphere.[17] The EEG pattern is helpful initially in the selection of an anticonvulsant medication and later to localize the site of onset and extent of seizure activity prior to surgery.

Functional imaging with PET indicates reduced metabolism of the brain adjacent to the leptomeningeal lesion but extending well beyond the area of abnormality depicted by computed tomography.[26] However, 2 of the 6 patients in this series with recent onset seizures had *increased* cerebral metabolism near the lesion. SPECT shows reduced perfusion of the affected brain.[27] Similar findings were recorded in an earlier study of regional cerebral blood flow using the xenon-133 inhalation method.[42] Nuclide scanning also shows reduced flow to the affected area in the dynamic phase of the test and localized increased uptake in the venocapillary phase.[43] While not all these studies are widely available, they may be of some use to initially establish a diagnosis and perhaps, in the case of PET and SPECT, in preparation for surgery.

Neuropathology

The leptomininges are thickened and discolored by increased vascularity. Microscopically these vessels are primarily thin-walled veins of variable size.[44,45] Some vessels are narrowed or occluded by hyalinization and subendothelial proliferation.[45,46] Angiomatous vessels sometimes extend into the superficial brain parenchyma, and the ipsilateral choroid plexus is often involved.[45] Microscopically abnormal vessels can be seen well beyond the lesion that is grossly visible.[44]

Cerebral atrophy, especially adjacent to the angioma, is typical. In some patients the atrophy becomes progressively more severe in early childhood before eventually stabilizing. Other children, particularly those with mild clinical features, may not develop visible atrophy at all. Microscopic features include neuronal loss and gliosis which, like the angioma itself, usually extend beyond the area of obvious abnormality.

The calcification seen radiographically is found in the outer cortical layers, occasionally extending into the white matter as well.[44,45] In younger children, calcium deposits are frequently noted in proximity to a vessel,[46,47] and some investigators believe that calcium deposits form within the vessel and later shift into the adjacent brain parenchyma.[44]

Treatment

Management of glaucoma and the cutaneous nevus is presented in other chapters; the discussion here will be limited to therapy of the neurologic manifestations of Sturge-Weber syndrome.

Epileptic seizures are usually the earliest and most challenging neurologic problem. Seizures in Sturge-Weber patients are notoriously refractory to medical management, but nevertheless many patients' seizures can be controlled with anticonvulsant medications combined with carefully monitored serum drug levels and attention to the optimum dosing schedule. A single drug regimen is usually more effective and better tolerated. Because of the focal or multifocal nature of Sturge-Weber syndrome, the seizures usually have a focal onset, although rapid secondary generalization of the seizure may make it difficult to confirm the localized onset. Carbamazepine is the drug most likely to be successful, especially when the seizures are clearly focal. Valproic acid is useful for generalized tonic-clonic seizures, myoclonic jerks, atonic seizures, and for the occasional patient with infantile spasms (ACTH is often used initially for infantile spasms). Phenytoin is effective as well, but the facial hirsutism and gingival hyperplasia often associated with its long-term use are particularly worrisome in patients who already have a cosmetically significant facial lesion. Barbiturates are better avoided if possible because of the frequency of behavioral disturbance and intellectual impairment (which are often then mistakenly attributed to the syndrome itself).

Treatment of seizures by hemispherectomy has been advocated for over 30 years.[48] Early hemispherectomy has been recommended for patients whose seizures began in infancy.[49] More recently, resection limited to the lobe predominantly affected has achieved good results,[19,50] and corpus callosum section may be a useful alternative for some patients.[51] Despite the general consensus that surgical resection is quite effective, there remains some debate about patient selection and the timing of surgery. Almost 1 patient in 5 has bilateral cerebral lesions, presumably limiting the surgical options unless one hemisphere is clearly causing most of the seizures. Although there are occasional exceptions, most physicians would not recommend surgery for a patient who has not yet developed seizures or for one whose seizures are fully controlled with medication. There is also understandable reluctance to initiate surgical resection of a portion of the brain that is functional and risk a new neurologic deficit—clearly in such a case the seizures have to be of such frequency and severity to justify the creation of a focal deficit that may well be permanent. Thus, surgery is usually reserved for patients with frequent, severe seizures, despite adequate medication trials, who already have clinical dysfunction of the area to be removed (e.g., hemiparesis or hemianopia). Limited resection is preferable to complete hemispherectomy, although the microscopic abnormalities often extend well beyond the area of grossly visible abnormality.

Prophylactic daily aspirin has been suggested as a means of preventing recurrent vascular thrombosis that may cause neurologic deterioration.[20,43,52] Although preliminary trials have been encouraging, controlled studies with aspirin present the same difficulties as with hemispherectomy. Until more information is available, routine use of aspirin cannot be enthusiastically endorsed. It does seem reasonable to use aspirin for patients with repeated clinical episodes suggesting transient ischemic attacks[20] and for patients with bihemispheric disease for whom surgery is not a reasonable option. Low-dose daily aspirin seems to be well tolerated in children,[53] although the optimum dose has not been clearly established.

Preliminary work by van Emde Boas and colleagues[54] suggests that propranolol reduces the frequency of episodic cerebral ischemia in Sturge-Weber patients whether or not they have clinical migraine. The authors suspect that vasospasm may account for episodic ischemia in some patients. Although their interpretation might seem more plausible if the vascular anomaly included more arterial changes, the observation is intriguing and deserves further study.

Summary

Sturge-Weber syndrome is characterized by a facial cutaneous angioma and a usually ipsilateral leptomeningeal angioma with abnormal cerebral venous drainage. Glaucoma is common. The clinical features include epileptic seizures, mental retardation, hemiparesis, hemianopia, or other focal neurologic deficits. The clinical profile is widely variable.

Radiographic findings include calcification in the cerebral cortex seen by computed tomography, and localized cerebral atrophy is typical of magnetic resonance imaging. The addition of magnetic contrast agents enables magnetic resonance imaging to outline the abnormal vessels of the leptomeninges and within the cerebrum. PET and SPECT scanning may also help to identify intracranial extension of the abnormal vasculature. Control of epileptic seizures with antiepileptic medications should be attempted; but if medication is unsuccessful, then surgical resection of the abnormal brain often controls the epilepsy. Surgery is not recommended in patients who are presymptomatic or those whose seizures are well controlled with medication.

References

1. Enjolras O, Riche MC, Merland JJ. Facial port-wine stains and Sturge-Weber syndrome. Pediatrics 76:48, 1985.
2. Roach ES. Diagnosis and management of neurocutaneous syndromes. Semin Neurol 8:83, 1988.

3. Roach ES. Congenital cutaneovascular syndromes. *In* Handbook of Clinical Neurology: Vascular Diseases. Volume 11. Edited by Vinken PV, Bruyn GW, Klawans HL. Amsterdam, Elsevier, 1989.
4. Tallman B, Tan OT, Morelli JG, et al. Location of port-wine stains and the likelihood of ophthalmic and/or central nervous system complications. Pediatrics 87:323, 1991.
5. Uram M, Zubillaga C. The cutaneous manifestations of Sturge-Weber syndrome. J Clin Neuroophthalmol 2:245, 1982.
6. Crosley CJ, Binet EF. Sturge-Weber syndrome. Clin Pediatr 17:606, 1978.
7. Ambrosetto P, Ambrosetto G, Michelucci R, et al. Sturge-Weber syndrome without port-wine facial nevus—report of 2 cases studied by CT. Childs Brain 10:387, 1983.
8. Taly AB, Nagaraja D, Shankar SK, et al. Sturge-Weber-Dimitre disease without facial nevus. Neurology 37:1063, 1987.
9. Gobbi G, Sorrenti G, Santucci M, et al. Epilepsy with bilateral occipital calcifications: a benign onset with progressive severity. Neurology 38:913, 1988.
10. Boltshauser E, Wilson J, Hoare RD. Sturge-Weber syndrome with bilateral intracranial calcification. J Neurol Neurosurg Psychiatry 39:429, 1976.
11. Bebin EM, Gomez MR. Prognosis in Sturge-Weber disease: comparison of unihemispheric and bihemispheric involvement. J Child Neurol 3:181, 1988.
12. Alexander GL, Norman RM. The Sturge-Weber Syndrome. Bristol, John Wright & Sons, 1960.
13. Meyer E. Neurocutaneous syndrome with excessive macrohydrocephalus (Sturge-Weber/Klippel-Trenaunay syndrome). Neuropaediatrie 10:67, 1979.
14. Kitahara T, Maki Y. A case of Sturge-Weber disease with epilepsy and intracranial calcification at the neonatal period. Eur Neurol 17:8, 1978.
15. Fukuyama Y, Tsuchiya S. A study on Sturge-Weber syndrome. Eur Neurol 18:194, 1979.
16. Welch K, Naheedy MH, Abroms IF, et al. Computed tomography of Sturge-Weber syndrome. J Comput Assist Tomogr 4:33, 1980.
17. Chevrie JJ, Specola N, Aicardi J. Secondary bilateral synchrony in unilateral pial angiomatosis: successful surgical management. J Neurol Neurosurg Psychiatry 51:663, 1988.
18. Peterman AF, Hayles AB, Dockerty MB, et al. Encephalotrigeminal angiomatosis (Sturge-Weber disease). JAMA 167:2169, 1958.
19. Aicardi J, Arzimanoglou A. Sturge-Weber syndrome. Int Pediatr 6:129, 1991.
20. Garcia JC, Roach ES, McLean WT. Recurrent thrombotic deterioration in the Sturge-Weber syndrome. Childs Brain 8:427, 1981.
21. Orr LS, Osher RH, Savino PJ. The syndrome of facial nevi, anomalous cerebral venous return, and hydrocephalus. Ann Neurol 3:316, 1978.
22. Fishman MA, Baram TZ. Megalencephaly due to impaired cerebral venous return in a Sturge-Weber variant syndrome. J Child Neurol 1:115, 1986.
23. Shapiro K, Shulman K. Facial nevi associated with anomalous venous return and hydrocephalus. J Neurosurg 45:20, 1976.
24. Anderson FH, Duncan GW. Sturge-Weber disease with subarachnoid hemorrhage. Stroke 5:509, 1974.
25. Cushing H. Cases of spontaneous intracranial hemorrhage associated with trigeminal nevi. JAMA 47:178, 1906.
26. Chugani HT, Mazziotta JC, Phelps ME. Sturge-Weber syndrome: a study of cerebral glucose utilization with positron emission tomography. J Pediatr 114:244, 1989.
27. Chiron C, Raynaud C, Tzourio N, et al. Regional cerebral blood flow by SPECT imaging in Sturge-Weber disease: an aid for diagnosis. J Neurol Neurosurg Psychiatry 52:1402, 1989.
28. DiChiro G, Lindgren E. Radiographic findings in 14 cases of Sturge-Weber syndrome. Acta Radiol 35:387, 1951.
29. Maki Y, Semba A. Computed tomography of Sturge-Weber disease. Childs Brain 5:51, 1979.
30. Enzmann DR, Hayward RW, Norman D, et al. Cranial computed tomographic scan appearance of Sturge-Weber disease: unusual presentation. Radiology 122:721, 1977.
31. Sperner J, Schmauser I, Bittner R, et al. MR-imaging findings in children with Sturge-Weber syndrome. Neuropediatrics 21:146, 1990.
32. Lipski S, Brunelle F, Aicardi J, et al. Gd-DOTA-enhanced MR imaging in two cases of Sturge-Weber syndrome. AJNR 11:690, 1990.
33. Elster AD, Chen MY. MR imaging of Sturge-Weber syndrome: role of gadopentetate dimeglumine and gradient-echo techniques. AJNR 11:685, 1990.
34. Furtado D, Rodrigues M. Pathogenie de la maladie de Sturge-Weber-Krabbe. Ann Med Psychol 105:398, 1947.
35. Hunt HB, Moore RC. Encephalo-trigeminal angiomatosis. Med Radiogr Photgr 27:53, 1951.
36. Poser CM, Taveras JM. Cerebral angiography in encephalo-trigeminal angiomatosis. Radiology 68:327, 1957.

37. Laur A. Cerebrales Riesenangiom mit Anomalie der grossen Arterien und multiplen sackformigen Aneurysmen. Dtsch Arch Klin Med 200:236, 1953.
38. Probst FP. Vascular morphology and angiographic flow patterns in Sturge-Weber angiomatosis. Neuroradiology 20:73, 1980.
39. Bentson JR, Wilson GH, Newton TH. Cerebral venous drainage pattern of the Sturge-Weber syndrome. Radiology 101:111, 1971.
40. Gabrielsen TO, Heinz ER. Spontaneous aseptic thrombosis of the superior sagittal sinus and cerebral veins. Am J Roentgenol Radium Ther Nucl Med 107:579, 1969.
41. Brenner RP, Sharbrough FW. Electroencephalographic evaluation in Sturge-Weber syndrome. Neurology 26:629, 1976.
42. Riela AR, Stump DA, Roach ES, et al. Regional cerebral blood flow characteristics of the Sturge-Weber syndrome. Pediatr Neurol 1:85, 1985.
43. McCaughan RA, Ouvrier RA, DeSilva K, et al. The value of the brain scan and cerebral arteriogram in the Sturge-Weber syndrome. Proc Aust Assoc Neurol 12:185, 1975.
44. Di Trapani G, Di Rocco C, Abbamondi AL, et al. Light microscopy and ultrastructural studies of Sturge-Weber disease. Childs Brain 9:23, 1982.
45. Wohlwill FJ, Yakovlev PI. Histopathology of meningofacial angiomatosis (Sturge-Weber's disease). J Neuropathol Exp Neurol 16:341, 1957.
46. Norman MG, Schoene WC. The ultrastructure of Sturge-Weber disease. Acta Neuropathol 37:199, 1977.
47. Roizen L, Gold G, Herman HH, Bonafede VI. Congenital vascular anomalies and their histopathology in Sturge-Weber-Dimitri syndrome. J Neuropathol Exp Neurol 18:75, 1959.
48. Falconer MA, Rushworth RG. Treatment of encephalotrigeminal angiomatosis (Sturge-Weber disease) by hemispherectomy. Arch Dis Child 35:433, 1960.
49. Hoffman HJ, Hendrick EB, Dennis M, et al. Hemispherectomy for Sturge-Weber syndrome. Childs Brain 5:233, 1979.
50. Rosen I, Salford L, Stark L. Sturge-Weber disease—neurophysiological evaluation of a case with secondary epileptogenesis, successfully treated with lobe-ectomy. Neuropediatrics 15:95, 1984.
51. Rappaport ZH. Corpus callosum section in the treatment of intractable seizures in the Sturge-Weber syndrome. Childs Nerv Syst 4:231, 1988.
52. Roach ES, Riela AR, McLean WT, et al. Aspirin therapy for Sturge-Weber syndrome. Ann Neurol 18:387, 1985.
53. Koerper MA, Addiego JE, deLorimier AA, et al. Use of aspirin and dipyridamole in children with platelet trapping syndromes. J Pediatr 102:311, 1983.
54. van Emde Boas W, Aicardi J, Barth P, et al. Therapeutic efficacy of antimigraine drugs in children with neurocutaneous vascular abnormalities presenting with transient ischemia. J Child Neurol 1:255, 1986.
55. Roach ES. Neurocutaneous syndromes. Pediatr Clin North Am (in press).

Chapter 10   Pulsed Dye Laser Treatment of Hemangiomas

Joseph G. Morelli
William L. Weston

Hemangiomas are the most common benign cutaneous tumor of infancy. They occur in approximately 3% of term newborns, with a somewhat higher incidence in premature infants.[1]

Hemangiomas have a well-defined natural history.[2,3] Most commonly, they are not present at birth and are first noted at 2 to 4 weeks of age. The presenting sign is usually a paling or light blue discoloration of the skin. Once the precursor lesion is present, hemangiomas enter a rapid-growth phase that lasts up to 9 months of age. During this period, the hemangioma grows at a much greater rate than the child. Between 6 months and a year, the rate of hemangioma growth slows and is roughly equivalent to the growth rate of the child. During the second year of life many hemangiomas begin to regress. The first sign of regression is central paling. This is followed by flattening of the lesion, and by 5 years of age 50% of hemangiomas have completely regressed.[2,3]

Regression defines disappearance of the vascular tumor, but does not necessarily imply return of the skin to a totally normal appearance. Frequently, excess slack skin, pigmentary alterations, and fibrofatty deposits remain following involution of the vascular component.[4] The residual skin changes are important when one begins to consider treatment options.

Because the natural history of most hemangiomas includes at least partial regression, and since most of the previous treatments had side effects that were potentially worse than no treatment, most authorities have recommended treating only those hemangiomas that had medical complications. These complications include high-output cardiac failure, localized clotting with consumption coagulopathy (Kasabach-Merritt syndrome), and obstruction of vital functions such as breathing, defecation, or urination.

Previous treatment strategies have included x-ray therapy, oral glucocorticosteroids, intralesional glucocorticosteroids, vessel sclerosis, electrocautery, surgery, and laser surgery.[5]

Initial lasers used for the treatment of hemangiomas included the carbon dioxide, argon, and the neodymium:YAG lasers. None of these lasers is selective for vascular lesions, and they all destroy tissue by the nonspecific production of localized heat, which destroys not only the tumor but also the surrounding normal skin. Secondary to the nonspecific thermal destruction of surrounding tissue, a significant degree of scarring was associated with these treatments.

The pulsed tunable dye laser at 585 nm (initially 577 nm) was developed for the selective destruction of the capillary-sized blood vessels of port-wine stains.[6–8] As previously discussed in depth in this text (see Chapters 2 and 4), the laser functions by targeting hemoglobin through the selection of the appropriate wavelength and then confining heat spread to the target tissue by optimizing pulse duration.[6] Although the laser was initially designed for treatment of port-wine stains, the blood vessels in hemangiomas approximate those of port-wine stains closely enough that the specificity of the pulsed tunable dye laser at 585 nm can be utilized to selectively treat hemangiomas. The laser has been FDA-approved for this indication, and many laser therapists have been treating hemangiomas with this laser.

Unlike the PWS treatment for which a significant amount of literature concerning optimal treatment parameters was published prior to the marketing of the laser, no such information existed for the treatment of hemangiomas. To date, only one article and two case reports have been published that detail the success of using the pulsed dye laser at 585 nm for the treatment of hemangiomas.[5,9,10] The largest study consists of a group of 10 patients. The laser treatment was beneficial in all patients, but 7 of the hemangiomas were treated after the beginning of involution and regression when most of the vascularity had already disappeared. Also, the lesions were not grouped according to depth of the hemangioma, a factor which is ultimately important in detailing the response of the lesion to treatment.

Because of the lack of information on the use of the pulsed dye laser at 585 nm for the treatment of hemangiomas, 6 obvious questions remain to be answered. These include: (1) in which cases are laser treatments truly beneficial; (2) if they are beneficial, what are the benefits; (3) what is the optimal age to begin treatment; (4) how frequently should treatments be performed; (5) what energy densities should be used; and (6) when should treatments be stopped?

In an attempt to answer as many of these questions as possible in as short a period as possible, a national multicenter study group has been formed. The study group has initiated laser treatment of hemangiomas by a standardized treatment protocol. To qualify for the study, the hemangiomas must have some superficial component; deep lesions are excluded as not amenable to treatment because of the minimal depth of penetration of the laser energy.[9] Children of any age may be treated, and it is hoped that the majority of children will be seen early, before the hemangiomas have entered into the rapid-growth phase. A starting energy of 6.0 J/cm^2 will be used and then adjusted according to outcome. Treatments will be performed every 10 to 17 days, until the lesions are gone or there have been two successive treatments that have been ineffective. Results will be judged by an independent panel of experts in pediatric dermatology. Because this study will take many years to complete, and because the literature contains only a few reports, much of the remainder of this chapter will be a discussion of our experience in treating hemangiomas at the University of Colorado School of Medicine Birthmark Treatment Center.

Treatment

Because the natural history and types of hemangioma vary markedly from those of port-wine stain, the goal of treatment is different, depending on the time at presentation for treatment and the type of hemangioma being treated.

The treatment times can be divided into the following categories: less than 3 months, or prior to the rapid-growth phase; during the rapid-growth phase (3–6 months); during the stable-growth phase (6–12 months); during regression (1–5 years); after maximal regression (>5 years).

The types of hemangioma treated can be categorized as superficial, mixed–predominantly superficial, mixed–predominantly deep, nodular, lip, ulcerated, and scarred lesions.

We have treated 55 patients and a total of 58 hemangiomas over the past 2 years. The age and type distribution are delineated in Table 10–1.

Superficial Hemangiomas

Superficial hemangiomas respond better to laser treatments than any other type of hemangioma. The main reason for this is that one of the shortcomings of pulsed dye laser treatment is its minimal depth of penetration. If the vascular abnormality is too deep, the laser cannot penetrate deeply enough with sufficient energy to cause specific vascular destruction. Superficial hemangiomas are usually only a few millimeters deep, and the laser energy can reach and destroy the majority of the vascular abnormality.

The optimal time for the treatment of superficial hemangiomas is immediately upon presentation. The initial superficial hemangioma is usually bluish to bright red and macular or minimally elevated, and thus it is theoretically possible to destroy much of the tumor before it has the opportunity to become more raised and to spread. For example, Glassberg et al.[5] first treated a child with a macular hemangioma at 6 days of age. Despite multiple complications from a subglottic component of the hemangioma, the child's skin was markedly improved at 4 months of age. This patient also received prednisone, which undoubtedly enhanced the lesion regression.

Although this is the optimal time for treatment of this type of hemangioma, because of the newness of the technique and the previous teaching to pediatricians and family practitioners, it is very difficult to get patient referrals at this time. Of the 55 patients that we have treated at the University of

Table 10–1. Age of Patients and Type of Hemangiomas Treated

Age (months)	<3	3–6	6–12	12–60	>60
Hemangioma type					
Superficial	3	9	3	4	1
Mixed	2	3	1	2	2
Nodular	3	2	0	2	2
Lip	0	2	2	3	1
Ulcerated	0	4	2	0	0
Scarred	0	1	1	3	1

Fig. 10–1. *A.* Three-month-old female before treatment. *B.* Two months later following 1 laser treatment.

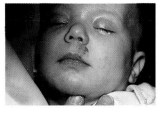 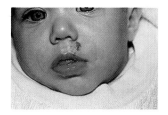

A   B

Colorado in the last two years, only 3 patients who have had superficial hemangiomas have been seen under 3 months of age.

The first patient had a very large superficial hemangioma similar in extent to the patient described by Glassberg et al.[5] She presented at 6 weeks of age with a rapidly expanding hemangioma that was already bright red and papular. She responded well to initial treatments, but unfortunately she developed subglottic stenosis with severe complications that eventually required tracheostomy. After this no further treatments were done, and the patient expired secondary to respiratory complications. The second patient presented at 1 month of age with a superficial hemangioma covering her entire left leg. She has been undergoing treatments for 4 months with excellent control of growth during the rapid-growth phase. The third patient was a 10-week-old female with a hemangioma under the nose that improved greater than 50% with a single treatment (Fig. 10–1).

Eleven patients with superficial hemangiomas presented during either the rapid- or stable-growth phase. Five of these patients had hemangiomas that were less than 3.0 cm^2 in total area. These patients received either 1 or 2 treatments; the treatments decreased the size of the lesion and prevented further growth. Because of the small size of these lesions and the stoppage of growth, no further treatments were undertaken. Three patients had hemangiomas greater than 20 cm^2 in size; these patients lived a significant distance away from the treatment center. One improved in a test area, but because of the distance the patient was unable to return for a further therapy. The other two improved by about 50% with two treatments (Fig. 10–2). Another three patients completed treatment with almost total clearance of the lesion before 15 months of age (Fig. 10–3)—this is years before expected clearance if no treatment had been performed. One of these patients, who is part of the national multicenter study, had only one half the lesion treated; there is an obvious difference between the treated and untreated portions (Fig. 10–4).

Fig. 10–2. *A.* Five-month-old male before treatment. *B.* Eight months later following 2 laser treatments.

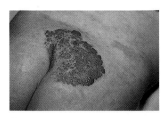 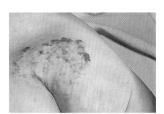

A   B

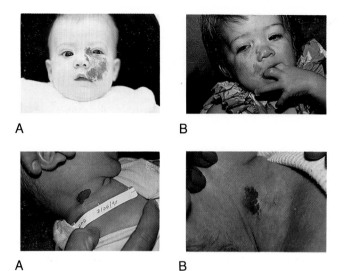

Fig. 10–3. *A.* Four-month-old female before treatment. *B.* Ten months later following 14 laser treatments.

Fig. 10–4. *A.* Two-month-old female before treatment. *B.* Four months later following 8 laser treatments to superior portion only.

Five patients with superficial hemangiomas presented while either in the regressive phase or after regression had ceased. These patients all improved or had total clearance of the vascular portion of the abnormality. At this time nothing could be done with the laser to change any damage to the skin caused by the expansive growth of the tumor (Figs. 10–5, 10–6).

None of the patients with superficial hemangiomas who were treated with the laser had an outcome worse than what would have occurred if the lesion had not been treated. All the lesions improved, with total clearance of the vascularity in some cases (Table 10–2). It is possible that more lesions could have been totally cleared with further treatment, but because the lesions were considerably smaller after initial treatments and had stopped growing, it was elected to discontinue treatments. Even the patients who began laser treatment after the tumor had entered the regressive phase had more rapid resolution of

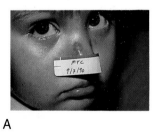
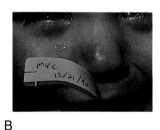

Fig. 10–5. *A.* Two-and-one-half-year-old female before treatment. *B.* Three months later following 6 laser treatments.

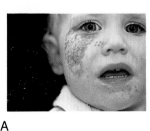
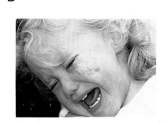

Fig. 10–6. *A.* Two-year-old white female before treatment. *B.* Eleven months later following 2 laser treatments.

Table 10–2. Outcome of Treated Hemangiomas

Age (months)	<3 C-I/T	3–6 C-I/T	6–12 C-I/T	12–60 C-I/T	>60 C-I/T
Hemangioma type					
Superficial	0-3/3	3-4/8	2-1/3	1-3/4	0-1/1
Mixed	0-3/3	0-3/3	0-2/2	0-1/1	0-2/2
Nodular	0-2/3	0-1/1	0-1/1	0-2/3	0-0/1
Lip	0-0/0	0-2/2	0-1/1	0-2/3	0-2/1
Ulcerated	0-0/0	0-4/4	0-2/2	0-0/0	0-0/0
Scarred	0-0/0	0-1/1	0-1/0	0-3/3	0-0/0

C=cleared   I–improved   T=total

the vascular component. Only one of the patients with a superficial hemangioma was treated at the optimal time, i.e., when the lesion first presents. This patient has done extremely well with control of the tumor by biweekly treatments. If patients present for treatment during the early macular phase of tumor development, we believe that many of the residual abnormalities following natural tumor growth and regression may be prevented.

Mixed Hemangiomas

Mixed hemangiomas contain both a superficial and deep component. They run a continuum from mostly superficial to mostly deep. The superficial components in general respond to laser treatment as if the deep component were not present. That is, when considering treatment goals, one can assume that the superficial hemangioma can be destroyed, but the deep component will be unaffected and will grow at its predetermined rate.

An exception to this rule is the nodular form, which is mostly raised above the skin level. We have treated 20 mixed hemangiomas (11 mostly superficial, 9 predominantly nodular). Mixed hemangiomas that are predominantly superficial respond similarly to those that are totally superficial (Table 10–2). Nodular hemangiomas follow a totally separate course. This type responds to laser treatment by initially developing signs of early regression. The first changes noted following treatment are a graying and paling of the bright red or blue color. Then flattening of the lesion begins. The amount of flattening that can be achieved by laser treatment depends on how raised the lesion was initially. The response of this type of hemangioma also depends on the age of the child when the treatments are begun. If treatments begin during the rapid-growth phase, the first change noted is a slowing or cessation of growth. This is then followed with subsequent treatments by graying and then flattening (Fig. 10–7). Lesions in which treatment begins after the rapid-growth phase, but which have not yet begun to regress, can be induced to enter a regressive phase. These lesions quickly become gray superficially (Fig. 10–8). They also slowly decrease in size. None of these lesions has been followed long enough to see if there is any long-term advantage of treatment versus no treatment. Hemangiomas in older children that have not regressed also respond only minimally to laser treatments. Thus, as with superficial lesions, the best results seen with treatment appear to be those which are treated before they have undergone maximal growth.

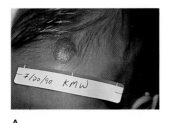
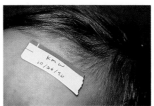

A   B

Fig. 10–7. A. Six-month-old female before treatment. **B.** Four months later following 9 laser treatments.

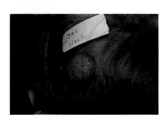
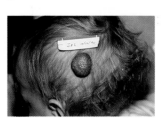

A   B

Fig. 10–8. A. Nine-month-old female before treatment. **B.** Two months later following 7 laser treatments.

Lip Hemangiomas

We have treated 8 patients who have hemangiomas of the lip. This type of hemangioma responds to treatment similarly to nodular hemangiomas (Table 10–2). That is, those treated during the rapid-growth phase cease growing and slowly begin to regress (Fig. 10–9). Those treated at a later stage show only a minimal response.

Ulcerated and Scarred Hemangiomas

Approximately 5 to 10% of hemangiomas ulcerate during the rapid-growth phase. The ulcerations often are slow to heal, are quite painful, and occasionally bleed. The mixed superficial and deep form of hemangioma is the type that most frequently ulcerates. We have treated 6 patients with ulcerated hemangiomas. In 3 of the 6 patients the ulcerations healed within 2 weeks following a single laser treatment (Fig. 10–10). The other ulcerations all healed following 2 or 3 laser treatments (Fig. 10–11). Pain was subjectively eliminated in all patients following a single treatment. The ulcerations that were less than 25 mm in maximal size healed with 1 treatment, while the larger ulcerations required the extra treatments. We

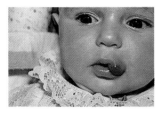
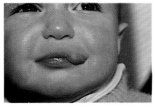

A   B

Fig. 10–9. A. Three-and-one-half-month-old female before treatment. **B.** Nine months later following 20 laser treatments.

Fig. 10–10. *A.* Five-month-old female before treatment. *B.* One month later following 2 laser treatments.

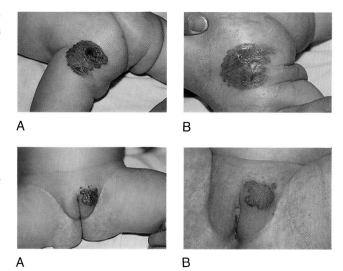

A   B

Fig. 10–11. *A.* Six-and-one-half-month-old female before treatment. *B.* One month later following 2 laser treatments.

A   B

believe that ulceration of hemangiomas is the best indication for laser treatment to date.

Unfortunately, many patients present for laser treatment after their hemangiomas have ulcerated and scarred. Despite this, we believe that it is not too late to perform the treatments. Such hemangiomas respond much like the mixed hemangiomas. Those with a superficial component respond well to the laser treatments. Treatments also help prevent recurrence of the ulcerations, and if done during the rapid-growth phase they minimize further growth.

Conclusion

The treatment of hemangiomas using vascular-specific pulsed dye lasers is in its infancy. There are only a few reports in the literature describing its effectiveness.[5,9,10] A multicenter study is currently under way to establish standard treatment protocols and to better define how the various types of hemangiomas respond to treatment and the time course of the response.

From our personal experience, the optimal time for treatment of any of the hemangiomas is at presentation, prior to the beginning of the rapid-growth phase. At this time all the various types of hemangiomas except the strictly deep form will respond to laser treatments by markedly decreasing the total growth of the tumor. Only a few of our patients have been available for treatment at the presentation of their hemangioma. Unfortunately, most of the patients are referred either during the rapid-growth phase or when their lesions have ulcerated and are not healing or are already scarred. Among our treated patients, the best results were obtained when treating those hemangiomas that have mostly a superficial component. Ulcerated hemangiomas responded to treatments with a rapid decrease in symptoms and healing within 2 to 4 weeks. Treatment of hemangiomas that contain more of a deep component may also be of benefit, but it will take more patients and followup time to establish the degree of benefit obtained.

References

1. Mulliken JB, Glowacki J. Hemangiomas and vascular malformations in infants and children: a classification based on endothelial characteristics. Plast Reconstr Surg 69:48, 1982.
2. Lister WA. The natural history of strawberry naevi. Lancet 1:1429, 1938.
3. Simpson JR. The natural history of cavernous haemangiomata. Lancet 2:1057, 1959.
4. Mulliken JB, Young A. Diagnosis and natural history of hemangiomas. *In* Vascular Birthmarks: Hemangiomas and Malformations. Edited by Mulliken JB, Young AE. Philadelphia, Saunders, 1988, pp 41–62.
5. Glassberg E, Lask G, Rabinowitz LG, et al. Capillary hemangiomas: case study of a novel laser treatment and a review of therapeutic options. J Dermatol Surg Oncol 15:1214, 1989.
6. Anderson RR, Parrish JA. Selective photothermolysis: precise microsurgery by selective absorption of pulsed radiation. Science 220:524, 1983.
7. Morelli JG, Tan OT, Garden J, et al. Pulsed dye laser (577nm) treatment of port wine stains. Laser Surg Med 6:1:94, 1989.
8. Tan OT, Sherwood K, Gilchrest BA. Treatment of children with port wine stains using the flashlamp-pulsed tunable dye laser. N Engl J Med 320:416, 1989.
9. Sherwood K, Tan OT. Treatment of a capillary hemangioma with the flashlamp pumped-dye laser. J Am Acad Dermatol 22:136, 1990.
10. Ashinoff R, Geronemus RG. Capillary hemangiomas and treatment with the flash lamp-pumped pulsed dye laser. Arch Dermatol 127:202, 1991.

Chapter 11   The Treatment of Cutaneous Hemangiomas of Infancy

John B. Mulliken

Anguished parents bring their perfect baby to you—now there is a rapidly growing vascular tumor on the face. The mother feels guilty. Was it something she did wrong? The parents want the birthmark erased. The bright red hemangioma seems to beckon you to do something, to try anything!

Over the centuries, physicians have demonstrated their resourcefulness in treating cutaneous hemangiomas. History teaches us lessons on how, and more often how not, to manage this most common tumor of infancy.

Historical Methods

In his 1714 treatise, Turner, the father of English dermatology, describes the use of caustics as well as surgical ligation and resection for hemangiomas.[1] The medical literature of the nineteenth century is replete with ingenious methods for garroting the blood supply to these most common tumors of infancy.[2] Subcutaneous ligation is still occasionally recommended by some authors.[3,4] Surgeons have also been willing to attempt extirpation of hemangiomas. Until the natural involution of hemangiomas was fully appreciated during the second half of this century, surgical excision was a primary mode of therapy.[5-7] A definite role exists for properly timed and well-planned surgical treatment of hemangiomas, as will be discussed later in this chapter.

There is an old observation that once a hemangioma ulcerated and healed, the scarred skin had a pale, almost normal color. It seemed logical, therefore, to induce ulceration in order to destroy cutaneous hemangiomas. Based on this syllogism, a litany of astringents, caustics, and refrigerants were applied to hemangiomas throughout the nineteenth century.[2] Another approach was intralesional injection of irritating solutions; this inaugurated sclerosant therapy. In the early part of this century, injection of boiling water became popular, thankfully for only a few years.[8,9] In the next era, hemangiomas were literally ''frozen to death,'' using carbon dioxide slush or solid crayon techniques.[10,11]

Hemangiomas have also been assailed with electromagnetic energy in various forms. Battery-powered electrolysis and thermocautery contrivances were the vogue in Victorian times. Modern thermocautery equipment with needlepoint attachment was used to puncture deep hemangiomas,[11] or for surface coagulation.[12] Radiation for hemangiomas reached its heyday during the middle of this century. Several modalities were employed, e.g., thorium-X varnish, interstitial gamma irradiation, radium/radon brass plaques, and low-voltage rays.[2] The proliferating hemangioma is, indeed, sensitive to even small doses of radiation. Today, radiation is well down the list of therapeutic alternatives because of the late skin complications, viz., atrophy, contracture, sclerosis, hypo/hyperpigmentation, telangiectasia, and permanent loss of hair from scalp, eyebrows, and eyelashes. By far the most damaging hazard of ionizing radiation for this benign disease is the late effect of radiation-induced malignancies. Furst and his colleagues studied cancer incidence in 18,000 patients treated with radiotherapy for hemangiomas in childhood and found a significantly increased risk of breast cancer, brain tumors, papillary thyroid cancer, and bone tumors.[12a]

Finally, compression therapy for hemangiomas deserves mention. Case reports of its success can be traced back to the nineteenth century; its history probably goes back even farther.[2] Yet, to date, there are no controlled prospective studies to validate compression. Any treatment protocol must take into account the fact that all hemangiomas spontaneously regress.

Current Management

Observation and Parental Support

Descriptions of spontaneous involution of hemangiomas can be found scattered throughout the medical literature of the last century. Nevertheless, appreciation for the natural course of hemangiomas remained clouded in confusion until 1938, the year Lister published his landmark paper.[13] Based on a carefully executed prospective study, Lister concluded that "no exception has been found to the rule that naevi which grow rapidly during the early months of life, subsequently retrogress and disappear of their own accord, on the average about the fifth year of life." Still, it took another 20 years before his findings were to be corroborated by other investigators.[14–20]

The majority of cutaneous hemangiomas do not require therapy. This does not mean, however, that nothing should be done. Foremost, the physician must sympathize with the parents' anguish. It is critical to listen to the parents' recounting of how the hemangioma appeared where once the child's skin was normal. A special effort must be made to dispel any blame, particularly the notion that the mother's behavior might have caused the hemangioma. The physician should explain that the cause of hemangioma is unknown, and he should briefly discuss what is known about the mechanism of angiogenesis. Possibly, conflicting ideas from relatives and other physicians might have to be resolved. Photographs and measurements should be taken during the initial visit so that subsequent changes in the lesion can be compared.

The parents may need repeated explanation of the benignity of this tumor. Hemangioma's progression and predictable involution are often effectively

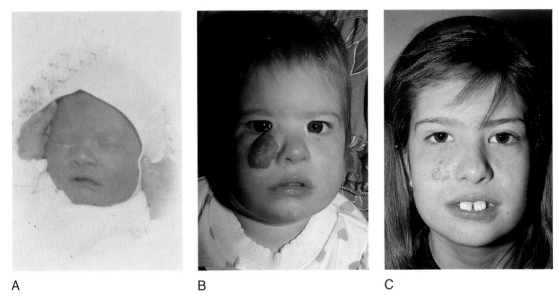

A   B   C

Fig. 11–1. Example of normal regression of superficial hemangioma. **A.** Photograph in newborn nursery reveals faint macular stain on the right cheek. **B.** The fully grown hemangioma is entering the involutive phase at 11 months. **C.** A few telangiectatic vessels remain at age 8 years—laser photocoagulation should be considered.

presented with the aid of textbook illustrations (Figs. 11–1, 11–2). Photographs of children with an involuted hemangioma, of similar size and location, are a welcome relief to the parents. The infant with a hemangioma should be seen as often as necessary to monitor the growth and to reassure the parents. More frequent visits are necessary when the hemangioma is either large, ulcerated, multiple, or located in a anatomically critical area. Needless to say, if the physician fails to gain the parents' confidence, they will search for help elsewhere. Once the hemangioma's growth seems to reach a plateau,

Fig. 11–2. Example of normal regression of deep hemangioma. **A.** Involutive-phase hemangioma on left cheek in a 6-year-old girl. See Fig. 1–4 in Chapter 1 of this text for an earlier stage. **B.** Regression is more obvious at age 8 years.

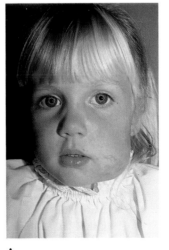 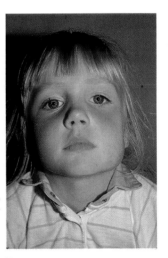

A   B

and the early signs of regression are obvious, the parents become more relaxed. Evaluations can proceed at 6-month to 1-year intervals.

Local Complications: Bleeding and Ulceration

Punctate bleeding from a florid cutaneous hemangioma is a frightening problem for the parents. They should be instructed how to compress the area with a clean pad, holding the pressure for 10 minutes by the clock. Repeated bleeding is rare. If it occurs, a mattress suture may be necessary. This sort of localized bleeding is usually not a manifestation of platelet-trapping coagulopathy.

The proliferating hemangioma may penetrate the overlying basement membrane. This manifests as ulceration and occurs in approximately 5% of hemangiomas.[21] Ulceration is more common for hemangiomas located in the lips and anogenital region. Secondary infection invariably accompanies ulceration. Very superficial ulceration responds to daily cleansing and topical antibiotic ointment application. Systemic antibiotics (based on culture results) are indicated only when there is evidence of cellulitis or systemic signs of septicemia. Recalcitrant ulceration is common. Wet-to-dry fine-mesh dressings may be necessary to debride the eschar. It often takes 2 to 3 weeks for an ulcerated hemangioma to heal by re-epithelialization. Once healed, there is a whitish patch of scar, in contrast to the surrounding red hemangioma (Fig. 11–3). Recurrent ulceration after healing is extremely rare. Extensive and/or refractory ulceration may be an indication for antiangiogenic therapy.

"Alarming" Complications

Certain hemangiomas, because of either their location or their behavior, give notice of approaching danger.

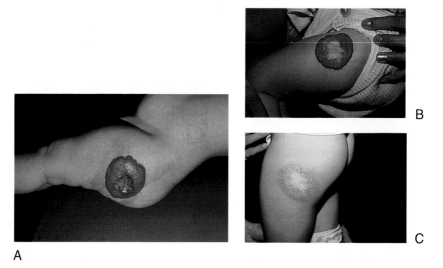

B

A

C

Fig. 11–3. *A.* Spontaneous ulceration of a thigh hemangioma. ***B.*** Healing by epithelialization leaves a pale central scar. ***C.*** Appearance following involution at age 7 years. The scarred central skin is not as normal as the surrounding skin that did not ulcerate.

Congestive Heart Failure With Visceral and Multiple Cutaneous Hemangiomas

Infants with multiple hemangiomas may present shortly after birth or several weeks later with a triad of congestive heart failure, hepatomegaly, and anemia.[22] The individual cutaneous hemangiomas are often quite small (5 to 10 mm diameter), dark red-purple in color, and hemispherical in shape. Subcutaneous hemangiomas and other more typical forms are also seen. The most common sites of visceral involvement are, in descending order, the liver, lungs, and gastrointestinal tract. Generalized hemangiomatosis occurs more commonly in girls, just as do cutaneous lesions.

The life-threatening complications are usually the result of hemangiomas within the liver. Hepatomegaly is often out of proportion to the degree of congestive heart failure. Less common presenting features are obstructive jaundice, intestinal obstruction, and portal hypertension.[23] Platelet-trapping coagulopathy may complicate hepatic hemangiomatosis, manifesting with petechiae and alimentary-tract hemorrhage.[24] High-output cardiac failure can also occur with large cutaneous hemangiomas in the absence of visceral hemangiomas.[25]

Although there is spontaneous regression of visceral hemangiomas, just as with cutaneous hemangiomas, the overall mortality rate is as high as 54%.[25a] Death is usually the result of congestive heart failure, infection, or hemorrhage.

Obstruction and/or Distortion

Visual. The proliferating hemangioma may impinge on or deform a critical anatomic structure. The best-known example is obstruction of the visual axis, causing deprivation amblyopia and failure to develop binocular vision.[26-28] Less well known is the fact that a hemangioma in the upper eyelid can distort the growing cornea, producing refractive errors, both astigmatic and myopic.[26] Anisometropia results in amblyopia. Even a small hemangioma in the upper eyelid can cause this mass effect. Frequent periodic refraction is mandatory. It is notable that even a large hemangioma in the lower eyelid or cheek is unlikely to cause visual disturbances. Hemangiomas may also cause strabismus, either paralytic (resulting from infiltration of the extraocular muscles) or secondary to the amblyopia.[27] Late complications of periorbital and adnexal hemangiomas include asymmetric refractive error, globe proptosis, blepharoptosis, and optic atrophy.

Respiratory. A hemangioma within the nasal tip may obstruct the vestibular passages. This can occur during the first 3 months of life when the infant is an obligatory nose breather. Usually, however, the obstruction is unilateral and the narrowing occurs slowly so that the infant adapts and breathes orally.

Far more insidious and life-threatening is hemangiomatous proliferation surrounding and impinging on the subglottic airway. About 50% of infants with subglottic hemangioma have a cutaneous lesion, usually in the cervicofacial region. The typical case scenario is an asymptomatic infant with all attention focused on a cutaneous hemangioma. By 6 to 8 weeks, pathognomonic biphasic stridor manifests, accompanied, in time, by respiratory distress. The typical clinical presentation is either a protracted episode of laryngotracheitis or recurrent bouts of "croup."[29] Any infant suspected of having a laryngeal hemangioma should have anteroposterior and lateral radiographs to assess the airway. The diagnosis is confirmed by direct laryngoscopy.

Auditory. Hemangiomatous proliferation in the parotid and auricular region may cause obstruction of the external auditory canal. Curiously, there is often bilateral involvement. This results in a mild to moderate conductive hearing loss. As the hemangioma regresses, blockage is relieved. There should be no permanent sequela unless bilateral obstruction persists beyond 1 year, when auditory conduction is necessary for development of normal speech.

Skeletal Distortion. Skeletal changes secondary to hemangioma are unusual. Deviation of the nasal pyramid, orbital enlargement, and minor indentation of the outer table of the calvaria can occur.[30] In these instances, the mechanism of skeletal distortion is presumed to be a mass effect on the nearby growing bone. More rare are cases of hypertrophy of the auricular framework or facial bones, documented in children with large hemifacial hemangiomas. Skeletal overgrowth may be secondary to increased blood flow to the tumor during the proliferative phase.

Platelet-Trapping Coagulopathy (Kasabach-Merritt Syndrome)

This hematologic complication of cutaneous hemangioma was first documented in 1940 by Kasabach and Merritt.[31] It occurs early in the postnatal and rapid-growth phase. The median age of admission to hospital is 5 weeks.[32] The hemangioma is either localized or diffuse. Characteristically the involved skin is deep red-purple, tense, and shiny. In large lesions, there may be a central area of softness, suggesting intralesional bleeding. Petechiae and ecchymoses are seen overlying and adjacent to the hemangioma. Subsequently, other skin areas become involved. Hematologic evaluation reveals a profound thrombocytopenia (from 40,000 to as low as 2,000 per cu mm). Early on in the proliferative phase, in addition to thrombocytopenia, there is a slightly low fibrinogen level. In time, fibrinogen falls to trace levels, while prothrombin (PT) and activated partial thromboplastin time (aPTT) become dangerously prolonged. There is the risk of acute hemorrhage (gastrointestinal, pleural, peritoneal, pulmonic, or central nervous system). There is also the hazard of a rapid increase in the size of the hemangioma (secondary to intralesional bleeding), causing compression of vital structures.

Skin Expansion

Some hemangiomas proliferate within the lower dermis and subcutaneous tissue layer with little involvement of the papillary dermis. These deep lesions, once labeled "cavernous" hemangiomas, predictably regress, leaving essentially normal skin. If the hemangioma proliferates in the superficial dermis, the skin becomes raised and finely bosselated with a vivid crimson color. The hemangioma, in effect, acts as a "tissue expander," destroying the normal collagenous-elastin framework of the dermis. With involution, the skin may be almost normal, or it may evidence variable atrophy with a few telangiectatic vessels. If the skin fails to contract, it will be loose, wrinkled, and slightly more pale than normal skin. Postregression, the once-protuberant hemangioma may "persist" as a noticeable fibrofatty tumor.

Biologic Therapy

The term "biologic therapy" specifies the use of a pharmacologic agent to control the proliferation of hemangioma and/or to initiate premature involution. Biologic therapy is indicated for an infant with: (1) multicentric or visceral hemangiomas causing high-output congestive heart failure; (2) a hemangioma that interferes with normal physiologic functions, e.g., breathing, vision, eating, or possibly hearing; (3) platelet-consumption coagulopathy; (4) a large lesion that distorts or expands soft tissues. Extensive and/or refractory ulceration is another possible indication for systemic therapy.

Chemotherapy

There are isolated accounts of the efficacy of chemotherapy for hemangiomas. In 1966, Rush reported use of intra-arterial nitrogen mustard for a large facial hemangioma.[33] More recently, cyclophosphamide was employed successfully in 3 infants with life-threatening pleuropericardial and liver hemangiomas.[34]

Steroid Therapy

In 1967, it was first reported that prednisolone resulted in accelerated involution in a consecutive series of 7 infants with "cavernous" hemangiomas.[35] This serendipitous finding was subsequently confirmed by others.[36–38] Clinically it was observed that a high dosage of corticosteroid was necessary. Oral administration was used initially. Soon thereafter, intralesional steroid was introduced in an effort to minimize the systemic effects.[39]

Mechanism of Action. The mechanism by which corticosteroid accelerates involution of hemangiomas is unknown. Edgerton hypothesized that steroid causes vasoconstriction and shrinkage of the vasculature within the hemangioma.[40] Another theory, proposed by Sasaki and Pang, is that high levels of exogenous corticosteroid suppress endogenous hormonal stimulation of hemangiomas.[41] Using a receptor assay system, these investigators demonstrated that hemangiomas contain increased estradiol binding sites. They present evidence that high levels of serum cortisone may inhibit the binding of estradiol to its receptor sites and thereby block estrogen-regulated proliferation.

The concept of "angiogenesis" and "antiangiogenesis," pioneered by Folkman and his coworkers, offers a productive pathway to pharmacologic control of hemangiomas.[42,43] The working hypothesis is that steroids modulate the control of endothelial proliferation. However, when cortisone was tested in the rabbit iris tumor model, there was no effect on angiogenesis, although inflammation was suppressed.[44] When heparin, which stimulates capillary endothelial migration in vitro, was given in combination with steroids, angiogenesis was inhibited.[45] Furthermore, cortisone and hydrocortisone, but not dexamethasone, are antiangiogenic in the presence of heparin and heparin fragments.[45] These findings are more intriguing, given the fact that mast cells, rich in heparin, are increased in proliferating hemangiomas.[46] Folkman and collaborators have also shown that certain tetrahydrocortisone analogs, those that lack glucocorticoid and mineralocorticoid activity, are the most potent "angiostatic" steroids.[47]

Administration. Once the decision to begin a trial of steroids is made, the drug should be promptly instituted. There is empirical evidence that the young proliferating hemangioma is far more responsive to steroid therapy than a mature lesion in a child over 1 year of age.[40] Systemic therapy is indicated for the complications of visceral hemangiomatosis, Kasabach-Merritt coagulopathy, or a large lesion causing distortion or obstruction. The usual dosage of prednisone is 2 to 3 mg/kg/day, given orally. Intravenous corticosteroid may be used in particular circumstances, e.g., for an infant with symptomatic sublgottic hemangioma. There is no evidence, however, that the response is better with intravenous than with oral administration. A sensitive hemangioma exhibits signs of responsiveness within several days to 1 week after initiating corticosteroid. The signs are obvious—lightening of color, softening, and diminished growth (Fig. 11–4). If there is no evidence of accelerated regression with 2 to 3 mg/kg prednisone per day, then the hemangioma will not respond to a higher dosage, and the drug should be

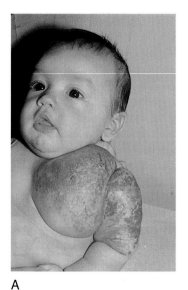
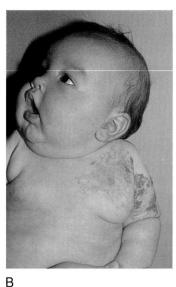
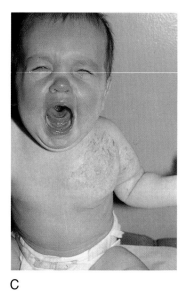

A   B   C

Fig. 11–4. *A.* Three-month-old infant with large hemangioma of the chest and arm; note skin expansion. *B.* Appearance at after 1 month on systemic prednisone, 2 mg/kg/day. Note remarkable response and Cushingoid facies. *C.* The infant at age 9½ months. Corticosteroids were discontinued one month earlier. The facial swelling has nearly disappeared, and the child is now growing at a normal rate.

Fig. 11–5. *A* and *B*. Four-month-old infant with extensive hemangioma of the face (with lip ulceration), with subglottic obstruction (requiring tracheostomy) and congestive heart failure. She was treated successfully with systemic steroids. *C* and *D*. Appearance at age 4 years: fine telangiectasias and fibrofatty residuum of lower lip.

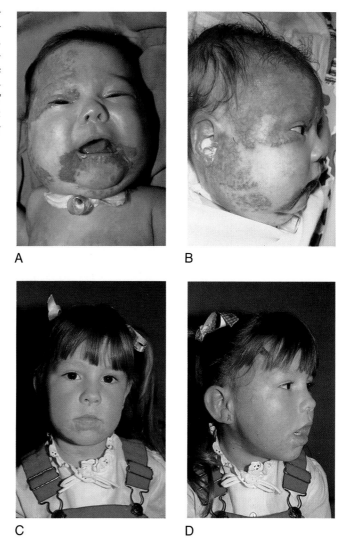

A   B

C   D

discontinued. If the hemangioma does respond, the dosage can be lowered slowly over several weeks. The duration and dosage of prednisone therapy depend on the tumor's sensitivity, location, and maturity. Rebound growth may occur in a proliferative-phase hemangioma at a low steroid level. In order to minimize regrowth, steroids have to be continued until involution is well under way, usually up to the time when the infant is 6 to 8 months old. Alternate-day administration is effective by this time, and the steroids can be slowly tapered and discontinued (Fig. 11–5).

Intralesional steroids should be considered for small protuberant hemangiomas in the face, and particularly for upper-eyelid lesions. The dosage is based on the child's weight and the size of the hemangioma. For periorbital lesions, Kushner recommends that each treatment should not exceed the injection of more than 40 mg triamcinolone acetate and 6 mg betamethasone.[48] Sloan and colleagues employed a similar regimen for hemangiomas which were located throughout the head and neck region.[49] No studies, however, document whether the additional betamethasone is more effective than triamcinolone alone. Usually a 27-gauge needle is used and several punctures are necessary to distribute the steroid throughout the lesion. Usually multiple injections (1–5) are necessary, spaced 6 weeks apart. Neither general nor local anesthesia is necessary.

Complications.   Very few complications are seen with a short-term, high-dosage course of steroids for hemangiomas of infancy. Gastritis, which happens infrequently, responds to antacid medication. Cushingoid facies often occurs, but resolves with a lower-dosage regimen or within a few weeks after discontinuation of steroids (Figs. 11–4B,C). Alternate-day therapy may minimize this well-known side effect. Some infants manifest diminished appetite and rate of growth. Once the steroids are stopped, however, the child resumes a normal pattern of weight gain. There are no reports of significant hypertension, salt/water retention, or long-term effects on skeletal maturation. Nevertheless, an infant on steroids is at increased risk for otitis media and pneumonia, as well as for overwhelming sepsis. It is advisable that the infant be followed closely by the pediatrician. The lowest effective dosage of steroid should be used for the shortest possible duration. Local steroids obviate systemic complications. However, cholestin plaque deposits and soft-tissue atrophy are seen as temporary problems.[48] Intralesional steroid injection for an eyelid hemangioma carries a potential vision-threatening risk for hematoma in the retrobulbar space; there is danger of accidental intraocular injection of depot steroid,[50] retinal artery occlusion, [51] and necrosis of the eyelid.[52] Hence, systemic steroids should be considered rather than intralesional injection for periorbital hemangiomatous infiltration.

Response Rate. The response rate for systemic steroid treatment of hemangiomas is reported in a range of 30[53] to 90%.[40] In the treatment of 23 infants with ''alarming'' hemangiomas, Enjolras and her colleagues report a varied responsiveness: excellent (30%), doubtful (40%), and total failure (30%).[54] Kushner notes a response rate of 60 to 80% with intralesional steroids for eyelid hemangiomas.[48] Sloan and colleagues, using the intralesional regimen, report 32% of hemangiomas showing greater than 50% reduction in volume and 32% with less than 50% reduction.[49] If these reports are taken in aggregate, the overall corticosteroid sensitivity for cutaneous lesions is about 50 to 60%.

There are no large studies of responsiveness in therapy of platelet-consumption coagulopathy. It appears to be about 50% of infants, perhaps less.[32,55]

When steroids are used in conjunction with other modalities for visceral hemangiomatosis, there is control of congestive heart failure in 60 to 70% of cases.[23,56–59] For steroid-resistant and life-threatening complications of hemangiomas, alpha-interferon and other antiangiogenic agents are being evaluated with clinical protocols.[60]

Embolic Therapy

Giant cutaneous hemangioma with platelet-trapping coagulopathy (Kasabach-Merritt syndrome) has been treated successfully with embolization via feeding arteries, using gelatin (Gelfoam) pellets[61] and polyvinyl alcohol

(Ivalon) particles.[62] Burrows and her coworkers report 7 instances of successful superselective embolization for hemangiomas obstructing vision or the airway.[63] Embolization has also been employed to control high-output congestive failure in hepatic hemangiomatosis.[62] The experienced Hôpital Lariboisiere group found "inconsistent results" with selective arterial embolization for "alarming" hemangiomas.[54] Embolization should probably not be considered unless there is a life-threatening complication and failure of response to corticosteroid therapy.

Surgical Therapy

Surgical excision is usually indicated for removal of fibrofatty residuum or skin laxity following complete regression of a hemangioma during childhood. Early in the evolution of these tumors, however, there are indications for operative intervention.

Surgery During Infancy

There are rare instances for operative treatment during the proliferative phase of the hemangioma life cycle. If a hemangioma is causing visual problems, and if it is nonresponsive to steroid therapy, excision (usually subtotal) may be indicated to relieve the pressure on the cornea (Fig. 11–6). Healy and coworkers publish a high rate of success with excision of obstructing subglottic hemangiomas using CO_2 laser.[64] There are reports of successful correction of severe thrombocytopenia following excision of a large cutaneous hemangioma.[65] Surgical excision should be considered if pharmacologic therapy is unsuccessful. For liver hemangiomatosis and congestive heart failure, unresponsive to steroids and embolization, hepatic arterial ligation has reported success.[23,66–68] Arterial ligation, however, is not always successful, as liver necrosis and abscess formation have occurred.[59]

Fig. 11–6. Operative therapy for a hemangioma in infancy. **A.** This infant's supraorbital hemangioma exhibited minimal response to intralesional steroid injection. There was pressure on the upper cornea, causing 1.5 diopters astigmatism. **B.** Astigmatism was corrected after excision of the hemangioma and patching of the opposite eye.

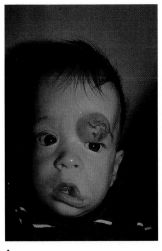
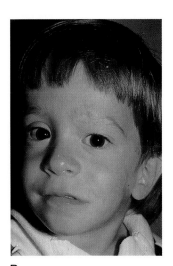

A   B

Surgery During Early Childhood (Preschool)

Parents rightfully will express their growing concern about a child with residual involuting hemangioma prior to entry into school. It is well documented that children begin to manifest a defined body or facial image around the age of 2 to 3 years. At this age language development allows the child to label objects. He may ask his parents about the birthmark or begin to refer to it by a name. The child may begin to manipulate the birthmark or indicate that he is different from other children. This is the time that child is exploring the world and his place in it, and perhaps his increasing attention to the birthmark is an indication of normal developmental self-awareness. These issues are, perhaps, best evaluated by a psychiatrist or psychologist before surgical excision is agreed upon.[69]

The child with an involutive-phase facial hemangioma is potentially vulnerable to psychosocial problems during school. Usually, however, the facial hemangioma is accepted by nursery school and kindergarten classmates. Problems are more likely to develop during first grade, when the child is exposed to older classmates. There are definite indications for subtotal or possibly total excision of an involuting hemangioma in early childhood.

The surgeon who undertakes excision at this stage must be cognizant of the natural history of hemangiomas and the basic principles of plastic surgery. As emphasized above, the indications for operative intervention are psychosocial. Yet excision is also anatomically reasonable if it is obvious that skin removal will be necessary in the future, because of color, quality, or contour, notwithstanding the final result of involution. Furthermore, certain anatomic regions are more likely to cause cosmetic problems, e.g., the nasal tip, glabella, and cheek. Some hemangiomas grow in a pendant fashion; even with complete involution, a bag of crepelike skin will remain. In such an instance, removal of the central section of the lesion corrects the contour. If there has been ulceration and scarring during infancy, it might be reasonable to begin serial excision of the scar during this time frame. The axis of excision should be parallel to the relaxed skin tension lines. Sometimes this is not possible because of the shape of the residual hemangioma. There are some instances where complete excision is both feasible and reasonable (Fig. 11–7). In general, subtotal, or staged, excision is the best approach. Caution is necessary so as not to overdo resection during this period for fear of causing late contour deficiency or deformity. Residual fibrofatty tissue and skin can always be removed, often with local anesthesia, when the child is older.

Following complete involution, a hemangioma within the lip often results in excess mucosal and submucosal tissue. Subtotal or contour excision is of benefit in these situations, and may be undertaken during early childhood. The nose is a psychologically sensitive focus. Also, nasal-tip hemangiomas seem to be slow to regress. They often leave a fibrofatty residuum with splayed underlying alar cartilages. Thomson believes that the results of natural involution of nasal-tip hemangiomas are better than those managed by excision.[70] When carefully considered, however, a definite role exists for subtotal excision to improve nasal contour. Nasal hemangiomas often are spheroidal, and there is a natural tendency to perform an external transverse and vertical wedge excision. A preferred technique is to enter the nasal tip either through a bilateral rim incision, an intercartilaginous incision, or via a

Fig. 11–7. Operative therapy for a hemangioma in early childhood. *A*. Three-year-old with a large involutive-phase hemangioma of the cheek. Although further regression was expected, expanded skin would remain. *B*. Skin excision was done at age 3 years; the girl is seen at age 9 years.

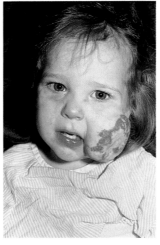
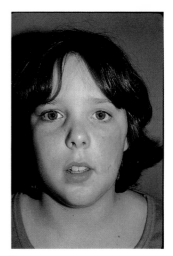

A   B

"low flying bird" external skin excision. The involuting hemangioma should be excised in three dimensions, and, if necessary, the alar genua should be apposed. Care should be taken not to remove too much hemangiomatous tissue, for with further involution a blunted nasal tip could result.

Surgery During Late Childhood and Adolescence

Usually it is best to wait until a child is 8 to 12 years of age before proceeding with removal of any excess fibrofatty tissue and skin that may remain after complete involution. Excision may be accomplished in single or multiple stages, always with respect for the relaxed skin tension lines (Fig. 11–8). A protrusive cutaneous hemangioma usually causes a tissue-expansion effect. Therefore, following regression, skin excision is usually possible without distortion of normal anatomic line and contour. If ulceration complicated the proliferative phase, the resultant hypo/hyperpigmented atrophic skin is best excised (Fig. 11–9). Usually, an excisional scar within the skin of an involuted hemangioma is remarkably well hidden.

Staged excision is a useful technique in dealing with circular-shaped, scarred, or hypo/hyperpigmented skin of the lip, cheeks, glabella, or scalp. If the overlying skin is nearly normal in color and elasticity, then excision from an intraoral approach is useful for residual hemangioma of the lip, cheek, or chin. In rare instances, where there is scarring and actual loss of skin, then use of custom-made tissue expanders is a useful reconstructive strategem. Blepharoplastic and rhytidoplastic types of skin excision are used to tighten the loose, crepelike skin that remains after involution of a large facial lesion. For the upper eyelid, excision of pretarsal and preseptal fibrofatty tissue, along with correction of blepharoptosis, is necessary. In rare instances, an ulcerated hemangioma may have destroyed a facial structure, e.g., helical rim, nasal-tip cartilage, or eyelid. These anatomic defects can be reconstructed with local tissue or by transferring tissue from a distant site.

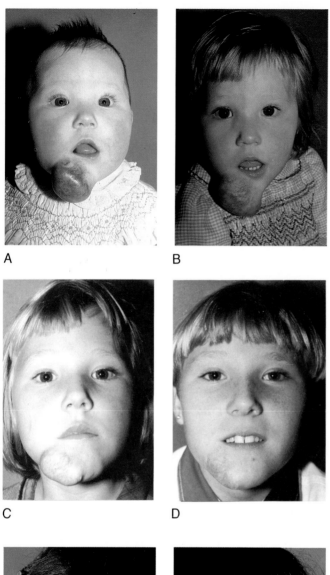

A   B

C   D

Fig. 11–8. Operative therapy for hemangioma in childhood. *A.* Large, protuberant hemangioma of chin in a 6-month-old infant. *B.* Regression underway at age 1½ years. *C.* Fibrofatty residuum at age 6 years. *D.* Age 9 years, following resection in two stages (age 6 and 7 years). The length of the scar and "dog-ears" are minimized by this strategem.

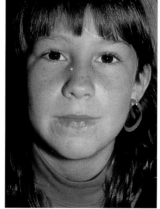

A   B

Fig. 11–9. Operative therapy for hemangioma in late childhood. *A.* Nine-year-old child, seen earlier in Fig. 11–5. She is bothered by crepelike skin, contour, and indistinct vermilion-cutaneous junction of her lower lip. *B.* Following excision of redundant skin and fat, placing scar along lip line.

Conclusion

Our attitude towards the treatment of cutaneous hemangiomas of infancy must be based on the knowledge that all these tumors invariably regress. Most hemangiomas are small; they grow and involute, causing minimal tissue alteration or psychologic disturbance to the child. Whatever the size of the hemangioma, the physician must fully appreciate the parents' distress and respond with appropriate support. In some instances, even small hemangiomas of the central face may cause problems for the family, and possibly for the child. In such situations, intervention is considered on an individual basis. Treatment should be undertaken always mindful of the dictum primum non nocere and with appreciation of the natural behavior of this tumor.[71]

Hemangiomas can also cause localized destruction, distortion, or obstruction of critical anatomic structures; or they may cause systemic complications, e.g., platelet consumption and congestive heart failure. For these problems, treatment is definitely indicated. Corticosteroid, either locally or systemically administered, is the most effective, currently available antiangiogenic drug. The response rate is in the 50 to 60% range. Prospective clinical trials with newer angiostatic agents are in progress.

Surgical extirpation, usually subtotal or contour excision, also has a role in the management of cutaneous hemangiomas. Operative strategems must be planned with a full appreciation of the particular hemangioma's growth pattern and a clear conception of the anatomic goal.

References

1. Turner D. De Morbis Cutaneis. A Treatise of Diseases Incident to the Skin. London, R. Bonwicke, W. Freeman, T. Goodwin, etc. 1714, pp 120–128.
2. Mulliken JB, Young AE. Vascular Birthmarks: Hemangiomas and Malformations. Philadelphia, W.B. Saunders, 1988.
3. Walsh TS, Jr. Giant strawberry nevi of the orbital arteries: treatment by ligation. Surgery 63:659, 1969.
4. Bingham HG. Predicting the course of congenital hemangioma. Plast Reconstr Surg 63:161, 1979.
5. Davis JS, Wilgis HE. The treatment of hemangiomata by excision. South Med J 27:283, 1934.
6. Matthews DN. Treatment of hemangiomata. Br J Plast Surg 6:83, 1953.
7. Modlin JJ. Capillary hemangiomas of the skin. Surgery 38:169, 1955.
8. Wyeth JA. The treatment of vascular tumors by the injection of water at a high temperature. JAMA 40:1778, 1903.
9. Reder F. Hemangioma and lymphangioma, their response to the injection of boiling water. Med Rec NY 98:519, 1920.
10. Semon HC. Treatment with the carbon dioxide snow pencil. Lancet 1:1167, 1934.
11. MacCollum DW. Treatment of hemangiomas. Am J Surg 29:32, 1935.
12. Matthews DN. Hemangiomata. Plast Reconstr Surg 41:528, 1968.
12a. Furst CJ, Lundell M, Holm LE, Silfversward C. Cancer incidence after radiotherapy for skin hemangioma: a retrospective cohort study in Sweden. J Natl Cancer Inst 80(17):1387, 1988.
13. Lister WA. The natural history of strawberry naevi. Lancet 1:1429, 1938.
14. Brain RT, Calnan CD. Vascular naevi and their treatment. Br J Dermatol 64:147, 1952.
15. Wallace HJ. The conservative treatment of hemangiomatous nevi. Br J Plast Surg 6:78, 1953.
16. Walter J. On the treatment of cavernous hemangioma with special reference to spontaneous regression. J Fac Radiol 5:134, 1953.

17. Ronchese F. The spontaneous involution of cutaneous vascular tumors. Am J Surg 86:376, 1953.
18. Blackfield HM, Torrey FA, Morris WJ, Low Beer BVA. The management of hemangioma. A plea for conservatism in infancy. Plast Reconstr Surg 20:38, 1957.
19. Simpson JR. Natural history of cavernous haemangiomata. Lancet 2:1057, 1959.
20. Bowers RE, Graham EA, Tomlinson KM. The natural history of the strawberry nevus. Arch Dermatol 82:667, 1960.
21. Margileth AM, Museles M. Cutaneous hemangiomas in children: diagnosis and conservative management. JAMA 194:523, 1965.
22. McLean RH, Moller JH, Warwick WJ, et al. Multinodular hemangiomatosis of the liver in infancy. Pediatrics 49:563, 1972.
23. Larcher VF, Howard ER, Mowat AP. Hepatic hemangiomata: diagnosis and management. Arch Dis Child 56:7, 1981.
24. Albert LI, Benisch B. Hemangioendothelioma of the liver associated with microangiopathic hemolytic anemia. Am J Med 48:624, 1970.
25. Stern JK, Wolf JE, Jr, Jarratt M. Benign neonatal hemangiomatosis. J Am Acad Dermatol 4:442, 1981.
25a. Berman B, Lim HWP: Concurrent cutaneous and hepatic hemangiomata in infancy: Report of a case and review of the literature. J Dermatol Surg Oncol 4:869, 1978.
26. Robb RM. Refractive errors associated with hemangiomas of the eyelids and orbit in infancy. Am J Ophthalmol 83:52, 1977.
27. Stigmar G, Crawford JS, Ward CM, et al. Ophthalmic sequelae of infantile hemangiomas of the eyelids and orbit. Am J Ophthalmol 83:806, 1978.
28. Haik BG, Jakobiec FA, Ellsworwth RM, Jones IS. Capillary hemangioma of the lids and orbit: an analysis of the clinical features and therapeutic results in 101 cases. Ophthalmology 86:760, 1979.
29. Healy GB, Fearon B, French R, McGill T. Treatment of subglottic hemangioma with carbon dioxide laser. Laryngoscope 90:809, 1980.
30. Boyd JB, Mulliken JB, Kaban LB, et al. Skeletal changes associated with vascular malformations. Plast Reconstr Surg 74:789, 1984.
31. Kasabach HH, Merritt KK. Capillary hemangioma with extensive purpura: report of a case. Am J Dis Child 59:1063, 1940.
32. Shim WKT. Hemangiomas of infancy complicated by thrombocytopenia. Am J Surg 116:896, 1968.
33. Rush BF, Jr. Treatment of a giant cutaneous hemangioma by intra-arterial injection of nitrogen mustard. Ann Surg 164:921, 1966.
34. Hurvitz CH, Alkalay AL, Sloninsky L, et al. Cyclophosphamide therapy in life-threatening vascular tumors. J Pediatr 109:360, 1986.
35. Zarem HA, Edgerton MT. Induced resolution of cavernous hemangiomas following prednisone therapy. Plast Reconstr Surg 39:76, 1967.
36. Fost NC, Esterly NB. Successful treatment of juvenile hemangiomas with prednisone. J Pediatr 72:351, 1968.
37. Brown SH, Jr, Neerhout RC, Fonkalsrud EW. Prednisone therapy in the management of large hemangiomas in infancy and children. Surgery 71:168, 1972.
38. Cohen SR, Wang CI. Steroid treatment of hemangioma of the head and neck in children. Ann Otol Rhinol Laryngol 81:584, 1972.
39. Azzolini A, Nouvenne R. Nuove prospettive nella terapia degli angiomi immaturi dell'infanzia, 115 lesioni trattate con infiltrazioni intralesionali di triamcinolone acetonide. Acta Bio-Medica 41:51, 1970.
40. Edgerton MT. The treatment of hemangiomas: with special reference to the role of steroid therapy. Ann Surg 183:517, 1976.
41. Sasaki GH, Pang CY, Wittliff JL. Pathogenesis and treatment of infant skin strawberry hemangiomas: clinical and in vitro studies of hormonal effects. Plast Reconstr Surg 73:359, 1984.
42. Folkman J. Angiogenesis. *In Thrombosis and Haemostasis.* Edited by Verstraete M, Vermylen J, Lijnen HR, Arnout J. Leuven, Leuven University Press, 1987, pp 583–596.
43. Folkman J, Klagsbrun M. Angiogenic factors. Science 235:442, 1987.
44. Gimbrone MA, Cotran RS, Folkman J. Human vascular endothelial cells in culture. J Cell Biol 60:673, 1974.
45. Folkman J, Langer R, Linhart RJ, et al. Angiogenesis inhibition and tumor regression caused by heparin or a heparin fragment in the presence of cortisone. Science 221:719, 1983.
46. Glowacki J, Mulliken JB. Mast cells in hemangiomas and vascular malformations. Pediatrics 70:48, 1982.
47. Crum R, Szabo S, Folkman J. A new class of steroids inhibits angiogenesis in the presence of heparin or a heparin fragment. Science 230:1375, 1985.
48. Kushner BJ. The treatment of periorbital infantile hemangioma with intralesional corticosteroids. Plast Reconstr Surg 76:517, 1985.

49. Sloan GM, Reinisch JF, Nichter LS, et al. Intralesional corticosteroid therapy for infantile hemangiomas. Plast Reconstr Surg 83:459, 1989.
50. Zinn KM. Iatrogenic intraocular injection of depot corticosteroid and its surgical removal using the pars plana approach. Ophthalmology 88:13, 1981.
51. Shorr N, Seiff SR. Central retinal artery occlusion associated with periocular corticosteroid injection for juvenile hemangioma. Ophthalmic Surg 17:229, 1986.
52. Sutula FC, Glover AT. Eyelid necrosis following intralesional corticosteroid injection for capillary hemangioma. Ophthalmic Surg 18:103, 1987.
53. Bartoshesky, LE, Bull M, Feingold M. Corticosteroid treatment of cutaneous hemangiomas: how effective? A report on 234 children. Clin Pediatr 17:625, 1978.
54. Enjolras O, Riché MC, Merland JJ, Escande JP. Management of alarming hemangiomas in infancy: a review of 25 cases. Pediatrics 85:491, 1990.
55. Esterly NB. Kasabach-Merritt syndrome in infants. J Am Acad Dermatol 8:513, 1983.
56. Braun P, Ducharme JC, Riopelle JL, Davignon A. Hemangiomatosis of the liver in infants. J Pediatr Surg 10:121, 1975.
57. Rocchini AP, Rosenthal A, Issenberg HJ, Nadas AS. Hepatic hemangioendotheliomata: hemodynamic observations and treatment. Pediatrics 57:131, 1976.
58. Clemmenson O. A case of multiple neonatal hemangiomatosis successfully treated by systemic corticosteroids. Dermatologica 159:495, 1979.
59. Pereyra R, Andrassy RJ, Mahour GH. Management of massive hepatic hemangiomas in infants and children: a review of 13 cases. Pediatrics 70:254, 1982.
60. Orchard PJ, Smith CM, Woods WG, et al. Treatment of haemangioendotheliomas with alpha interferon. Lancet 2:565, 1989.
61. Argenta LC, Bishop E, Cho KJ, et al. Complete resolution of life-threatening hemangioma by embolization and corticosteroids. Plast Reconstr Surg 760:739, 1982.
62. Stanley P, Gomperts E, Woolley MM. Kasabach-Merritt syndrome treated by therapeutic embolization with polyvinyl alcohol. Am J Pediatr Hematol Oncol 8:308, 1986.
63. Burrows PE, Lasjaunias PL, TerBrugge KG, Flodmark O. Urgent and emergent embolization of lesions of the head and neck in children: indications and results. Pediatrics 80:386, 1987.
64. Healy G, McGill T, Friedman EM. Carbon dioxide laser in subglottic hemangioma. An update. Ann Otol Rhinol Laryngol 93:370, 1984.
65. Hill GL, Longino LA. Giant hemangioma with thrombocytopenia. Surg Gynecol Obstet 114:304, 1962.
66. DeLorimier AA, Simpson EB, Baum RS, Carlsson E. Hepatic artery ligation for hepatic hemangiomatosis. N Engl J Med 277:333, 1967.
67. Keller L, Bluhm JF. Diffuse neonatal hemangiomatosis; a case with heart failure and thrombocytopenia. Cutis 23:295, 1979.
68. Shannon K, Buchanan GR, Votteler TP. Multiple hepatic hemangiomas: failure of corticosteroid therapy and successful hepatic artery ligation. Am J Dis Child 36:275, 1982.
69. Harrison AM. The emotional impact of a vascular birthmark. In *Vascular Birthmarks: Hemangiomas and Malformations*. Edited by Mulliken JB, Young AE. Philadelphia, W.B. Saunders, 1988, 454–462.
70. Thomson HG, Lanigan J. The Cyrano nose—a clinical review of hemangioma of the nasal tip. Plast Reconstr Surg 63:155, 1979.
71. Mulliken JB. A plea for a biologic approach to hemangiomas of infancy. Arch Dermatol 127:243, 1991.

Chapter 12   Noncongenital Benign Cutaneous Vascular Lesions: Pulsed Dye Laser Treatment

Oon Tian Tan
Amal K. Kurban

Benign cutaneous vascular lesions commonly present for laser treatment. Unlike port-wine stain (PWS), hemangioma, and a few cases of essential telangiectasia, most lesions are small, discrete, and with the abnormal vessels located in the superficial dermis. Hence, treatment of these noncongenital lesions can often be performed in the office using treatment modalities such as electrocautery and a variety of lasers (Table 12–1).

In general, the cosmetic results following electrocautery have been satisfactory. The question of why time and effort should be invested in considering other treatment modalities if the lesions can be easily removed using electrocautery then arises. As has been well established, the fundamental problem arising from injury induced by any thermal source such as electrocautery is the lack of specificity of the injury. Delivery of heat of unspecified intensity and duration often results in nonspecific injury of all

Table 12–1. Treatment Modalities Used for Removing Benign Cutaneous Vascular Lesions

Electrocautery
Lasers
- Carbon dioxide
- Neodymium:YAG
- Argon
- Argon pumped dye (577 nm)
- Pulsed dye (577/585 nm)
- Copper vapor (578 nm)

**Table 12–2. Noncongenital Benign
Cutaneous Vascular
Lesions Treated Using
the Pulsed Dye Laser**

Macular Lesions (Telangiectasia)
- Essential
    localized
    generalized
- Rosacea
- CREST syndrome
- Poikiloderma of Civatte
- Post–procedure/trauma
    x-irradiation
    skin graft
    trauma
    sclerotherapy
- Arborizing telangiectasia of lower limbs

Papular Lesions
- Spider angioma
- Tufted angioma (angioblastoma)
- Hereditary hemorrhagic telangiectasia
- Angiokeratoma
- Pyogenic granuloma
- Angiofibroma (adenoma sebaceum)
- Blue rubber bleb syndrome
- Venous lake
- Lymphangioma

tissues at the exposed site. Such widespread injury heals by scar formation, which is often accompanied by alteration in skin pigmentation (both hypo- and hyperpigmentation).

Such adverse effects have been of little consequence when lesions are small, single, and discrete. Even if pinpoint hypopigmented scars result from the various nonspecific treatments, patients have, in general, found them cosmetically acceptable. Difficulties have arisen, however, when the abnormal vessels are distributed over large areas, and/or when the lesions have recurred, requiring multiple, repeated treatments to clear them.

As with the treatment of PWS, discussed in Chapters 6 and 7, lasers (Table 12–1) have been successfully used to treat different types of benign cutaneous vascular lesions (Table 12–2). Treatment of many of these disease entities will be discussed individually in this chapter.

Laser Treatments of Benign Cutaneous Vascular Lesions

A variety of laser parameters has been used to treat benign cutaneous vascular lesions.[1–6] Of these, the spot size of the laser has been the parameter most commonly altered for clinical application (Table 12–3). The reason

Table 12–3. Laser Parameters Used To Treat Benign Cutaneous Vascular Lesions

Laser	Wavelength (nm)	Spotsize
Argon	488/514	100 μm, 1 mm
Argon	577	100 μm
Pumped dye	577/585	1 mm
Pulsed dye	577/585	3 & 5 mm
Copper vapor	578	1 & 3 mm
Nd:YAG	1,600	200 μm, 1–3 mm
CO_2	10,600	1 mm

most often given for changing the spot size, usually to less than 1 mm, has been the need to minimize both the acute and the post-treatment skin-color changes following laser irradiation. Unlike those with PWS, most patients seeking treatment of their benign cutaneous vascular lesions prefer to have their skin appear as ''normal'' as possible immediately following laser treatment. This seems to be a major cosmetic concern of these patients, partly because most lesions presenting for treatment are in visible sites.

The effects on tissues of different combinations of laser parameters such as spotsize have only recently been appreciated.[7,8] As has been clearly discussed in Chapter 2, the correct combination of laser parameters controls the degree and extent of injury induced at the laser-exposed site. A change in the spotsize diameter has been shown to affect not only the depth of penetration of the laser beam but also the degree of injury induced in the tissues of the laser-irradiated site.[7,8]

Besides spot size, wavelength and pulse duration have also been demonstrated to affect specificity of injury (see Chapter 2). In the case of superficial cutaneous blood vessels, lasers tuned to 577/585 nm over a pulse duration of 300 to 500 μsec have been shown to selectively destroy these vessels. Their application for the treatment of some benign cutaneous vascular lesions, as outlined in Table 12–2, has not only resulted in clearance of these lesions but also left the treated areas indistinguishable from normal adjacent skin.[9–12] Details of treatment parameters needed for removing these benign cutaneous vascular lesions will be discussed below.

Macular Lesions (Telangiectasia)

Telangiectatic lesions can present in several ways. They can be: (a) small, individual clusters localized in certain parts of the body; (b) more extensive and more widespread, involving large areas of skin such as the ''butterfly'' distribution of the face; or (c) progressive and widespread, involving large areas or even the whole body, as may be the case with generalized essential telangiectasia.

Fig. 12–1. *A.* Actinically induced facial telangiectasia prior to laser treatment. *B.* Post–pulsed dye laser facial telangiectasia. Note that the treated skin is indistinguishable from normal adjacent skin.

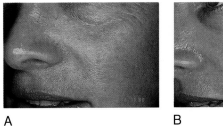
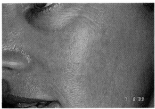

A   B

Essential Telangiectasia

Localized

Actinic. Actinically induced telangiectasia is probably the most common type presenting for laser treatment in the Caucasian population (Fig. 12–1A). Unless previously treated by other treatment modalities such as electrocautery, most respond to a single treatment using the pulsed dye laser at 577/585 nm over a pulse duration of 300 to 500 μsec (Fig. 12–1B). Treatment is generally simple, involving 1 or 2 exposures at each site at fluences of between 6.0 and 6.25 J/cm². An adverse effect that may be encountered (most commonly where the telangiectasia is more widespread) is transient hyperpigmentation. This often fades over time, usually between 3 to 6 months.

In those patients who have undergone previous treatments using electrocautery or CW lasers, further treatment of the facial telangiectasia and erythema using the pulsed dye laser may unmask the scarring (hypopigmentation and depression) induced by previous treatment modalities. Therefore, it is advisable to warn those patients who fall into this category that there could likely be sequelae.

Besides these, pulsed dye laser treatments of actinically induced telangiectasia are simple to perform, and patients have been delighted with the cosmetic results (Fig. 12–1).

Generalized

Generalized essential telangiectasia most commonly occurs in females.[13,14] It can present at any time from just before puberty to middle age. The condition often starts as isolated ''patches'' of telangiectasia most commonly in the lower limbs, gradually spreading upwards as extensive telangiectatic sheets over the rest of the body, with the exception of the palms, soles, and mucous membranes (Fig. 12–2A,D). This takes several years to occur. Those affected by generalized essential telangiectasia appear to be otherwise well and do not have any evidence of systemic problems.

This entity was initially described by Hutchinson in 1889[15] and given the nomenclature generalized essential telangiectasia by Radcliffe-Crocker in 1893.[16] After its introduction into the literature, many different disease entities were included under this classification, causing great confusion. In attempts to prevent further confusion, the term generalized essential

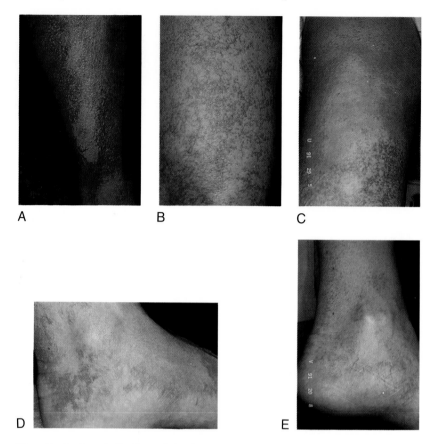

Fig. 12–2. *A* and ***B*.** Essential telangiectasia involving the lower leg prior to treatment. ***C*.** Part of the leg after treatment using the pulsed dye laser. Note that the skin is normal in color and texture when compared to adjacent normal skin. ***D*.** Pretreated essential telangiectasia on the foot. This appears to be a typical site for these lesions. ***E*.** The same foot cleared of the telangiectasia after one laser treatment.

telangiectasia is now reserved to describe only this acquired, apparently benign, vascular condition.[13,14]

Although the disease itself appears to be of no consequence, the lesions are widespread and unsightly. It is for this reason that patients seek treatment. Until recently, treatments have generally been unhelpful, with the exception according to one report that oral tetracycline for three months was helpful.[17] More recently, the pulsed dye laser has been used effectively to treat these lesions at fluences of around 6.0 J/cm^2 over pulse durations of between 300 and 500 μsec (Fig. 12–2B,C,E). The treated skin, cleared of the telangiectasia, appears normal in color and texture.

Rosacea

Rosacea, commonly presenting for treatment with widespread telangiectasia, affects middle-aged men and women. Other manifestations of rosacea include pustules, erythematous plaques, and hypertrophy of particular parts of the face (Fig. 12–3) such as the nose (rhinophyma).

Patients with rosacea present for treatment because of progressive telangiectasia and persistent erythema as well as pustules. Oral antibiotics,

Fig. 12–3. **A.** Telangiectasia and erythema on the nose and malar regions associated with rosacea. **B.** Post–pulsed dye laser treatment of the same areas.

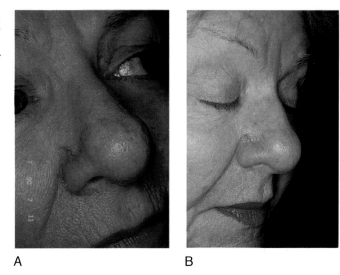

A   B

e.g., tetracycline or minocycline, as well as topical treatments (e.g., Metrogel) are routinely prescribed for treatment of rosacea. Although this combination treatment controls many of the major symptoms, other treatment modalities such as lasers are needed to clear the telangiectasia and erythema, which are an integral part of this syndrome (Fig. 12–3).

Because the pathogenesis and causal mechanism of rosacea remain obscure, it is not known how the pulsed dye laser treatment affects the disease process, and whether laser treatments will, in any way, influence the progression and chronicity of the rosacea. Anecdotally, patients with rosacea treated with the pulsed dye laser at 577/585 nm at fluences of around 6.0 to 6.5 J/cm^2 have reported symptomatic relief of their skin condition. Not only have pulsed dye laser treatments improved the telangiectasia and facial erythema, but several patients have also reported that with progressive laser treatments the number and frequency of pustules have decreased, enabling some of them to curtail or even stop systemic antibiotics altogether.

CREST Syndrome

CREST is the acronym for *C*alcinosis, *R*aynaud's phenomenon, *e*sophageal, *s*cleroderma, and *t*elangiectasia. Patients with this syndrome often present for laser treatment because of telangiectasia involving large areas of their skin and mucous membranes (Fig. 12–4A). Unlike the other types of telangiectasia discussed, those associated with CREST appear as 2 to 4 mm matted telangiectasia without a central arteriole and tend to be less responsive to conventional treatment such as electrocautery. Other clinical problems unique to this syndrome are poor cutaneous circulation and sclerodermoid changes associated with poor wound healing. Therefore, when a suitable treatment modality for removing telangiectases in CREST is evaluated, the severity and extent of injury induced at each treatment site are important considerations. The ideal treatment modality should be one in which the injury is localized only to abnormal vessels, with minimal injury induced in healthy adjacent structures such as epidermis and dermal collagen. This would

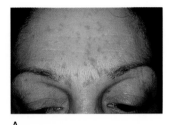
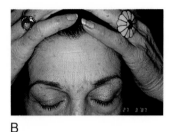

A   B

Fig. 12–4. *A.* Pretreated telang-iectasia associated with CREST. ***B.*** Post–pulsed dye laser treatment of these vessels.

reduce the risk of wound infection and would be an added therapeutic advantage.

Therefore, because of the problems unique to CREST, the pulsed dye laser emitting at 577/585 nm over a pulse duration of between 300 and 500 μsec and a 5 mm diameter spotsize has been an appropriate and effective modality for treating these lesions (Fig. 12–4B). Of significance has been the fact that the treated sites have healed without scar formation. Scarring has not occurred even after several laser exposures to the same site. Multiple retreatments seem to be required for clearing CREST telangiectasia.

Poikiloderma of Civatte

Poikiloderma of Civatte is a common condition, affecting women more than men, especially those with a long history of sun exposure. The sides of the neck are usually affected, appearing erythematous, finely wrinkled, and hyperpigmented (Fig. 12–5A). Histologically, there is atrophy and hyper-pigmentation of the epidermis in addition to the presence of ectatic vessels in the upper dermis.

Because of the location of the lesion and the discoloration which accompanies it, patients seek treatment to clear the erythematous as well as the hyperpigmented components of this condition. The pulsed dye laser, at 585 nm at around 6.0 J/cm^2, has effectively cleared the telangiectasia, leaving the laser-irradiated skin appearing normal in color and texture (Fig. 12–5B). The clearance of the erythema and telangiectasia in the absence of scar formation has been of paramount importance, especially in an anatomic area where scarring can be particularly problematic.

Post–Procedure/Trauma

Post–x-irradiation. Telangiectasia can occur in skin following exposure to x-ray irradiation. Because the vessels tend to be superficial, they have been reported to respond well to the pulsed dye laser system.

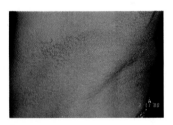
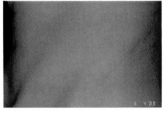

A   B

Fig. 12–5. *A.* Poikiloderma of Civatte on the neck prior to laser treatment. Note that the skin is erythematous as well as hyperpig-mented. ***B.*** Clearance of the ery-thema and telangiectasia following pulsed dye laser treatment. Note that the treated skin is as normal as uninvolved adjacent skin.

Fig. 12–6. *A*. Pretreated, post–skin graft telangiectasia. ***B*.** Post–pulsed dye laser treated, post–skin graft telangiectasia. Note that the laser treatment has not affected the architecture of the graft.

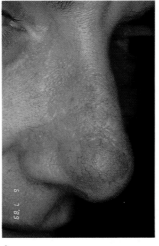 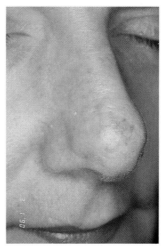

A   B

Post–skin graft. Telangiectasia can occur and be problematic after a successful skin graft especially in areas such as the face (Fig. 12–6A).

In treating postgraft telangiectasia, it is important that (a) the induced injury be localized only to the abnormal vessels, and that (b) injury to adjacent healthy structures be minimized, so that the graft or underlying disorder for which the surgery and graft were performed remains intact. If both these conditions can be achieved, any complications which might arise from additional scar formation should be minimized.

The pulsed dye laser will effectively clear the telangiectasia without adversely affecting the architecture of the graft or the underlying tissues. As is evident in Figure 12–6, this laser will selectively and effectively clear the postgraft telangiectasia without adversely altering the grafted site (Fig. 12–6B).

Post-trauma. Telangiectasia can occur at sites which either have been traumatized or have been constantly irritated by physical and/or chemical irritants (Fig. 12–7A). Because the telangiectatic vessels in most instances appear to be superficial, they have responded well to the pulsed dye laser when they have been exposed to fluences of around 6.0 J/cm^2 (Fig. 12–7B).

Postsclerotherapy. There have been recent reports of the appearance of fine telangiectatic vessels around sites where sclerotherapy was previously performed in the lower limbs. The history of preceding sclerotherapy and the localization of the telangiectasia to the treated areas are diagnostic.

Fig. 12–7. *A*. Telangiectasia on the upper lip induced by constant trauma to the area. ***B*.** The upper lip following pulsed dye laser treatment.

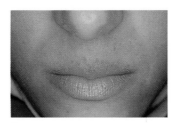 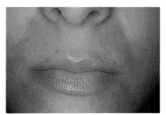

A   B

Arborizing Telangiectasia of the Lower Limbs

The treatment and management of these lesions are discussed in detail in Chapter 13.

Papular Lesions

Spider Angioma

Spider angiomata (nevus araneus), characterized by an elevated central papule from which capillaries radiate, commonly present for treatment in adults as well as in children (Fig. 12–8A). Spider angiomas are frequent both in pregnancy and liver cirrhosis. These lesions are palpable and can occasionally be pulsatile. The upper trunk and face are the usual sites, the latter being particularly common.

Histologically, there is a central artery with radiating branches. These lesions respond well to the pulsed dye laser at fluences of around 6.0 J/cm^2 using a 5 mm diameter spotsize (Fig. 12–8B). Because the lesions generally are small, only a single treatment is required to clear them. Most treated areas heal, leaving the treated sites indistinguishable in color and texture from normal adjacent skin (Fig. 12–8B).

Tufted Angioma (Angioblastoma)

Tufted angioma is a distinct, benign, unusual form of acquired vascular proliferation most commonly occurring in the neck and upper trunk regions of young people.[18] The majority of lesions have occurred in patients under 5 years old, although a few individuals have developed lesions as late as the fourth, fifth, and even sixth decades of life.[19]

Tufted angiomas differ from other forms of vascular proliferation by possessing distinct histopathologic features characterized by the presence of hypertrophied endothelial cells scattered throughout the dermis. The striking feature on light microscopy is the "cannonball" distribution of the vessels, which are composed of tightly packed capillary vessels occurring in "discrete or ovoid tufts" against a background of normal, unaffected dermal collagen.[21] Examination of these ovoid tufts on high magnification aided by the use of special stains (such as reticulin stains) reveals that the vascular tufts appear to be composed of hypertrophied endothelial cells packed together

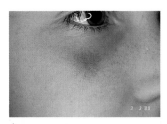 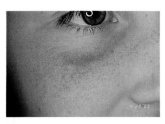

Fig. 12–8. *A.* Pretreated angioma. *B.* Post–pulsed dye laser treated angioma. Note that the skin appears normal.

A   B

with capillary lumen.[21] In none of the histopathologic specimens examined was there any evidence of malignant transformation.

The clinical course of tufted angioma is often slow, with the lesions developing insidiously over several years before growth ceases completely. However, rapid growth of these angiomas, developing over several months, has also been reported.[20]

Hereditary Hemorrhagic Telangiectasia

Hereditary hemorrhagic telangiectasia (HHT), an autosomal dominant disorder, is characterized by multiple telangiectasias of the nasal and oral cavities. The abnormal ectatic thin-walled veinlike vessels lie beneath the epithelial surface.[22] These vascular abnormalities can also be found in the skin, gastrointestinal tract, central nervous system, and respiratory system.

The cutaneous telangiectasia associated with HHT has been responsive to 577/585 nm pulsed dye laser treatments when exposed to fluences of around 6.0 J/cm^2. However, a common problem associated with this condition is epistaxis, which is progressive and can be frequent and often severe. The nose bleeds can incapacitate the patient in the early and middle stages of the disease, restricting employability and activities. The disease progressively worsens to the point when the bleeding is so severe and frequent that repeated blood transfusions may be required. At this stage, the end stage of the disease, arterial ligation and embolization may be needed. In spite of these, sustained improvement is not achieved. Nasal mucosa stripping with skin grafting is also often performed at this stage, even though recurrence is inevitable because of the ability of these vessels to repopulate the new skin graft.[22] Systemic hormonal therapy with estrogen and progesterone has been reported to decrease the frequency and severity of the epistaxis.[24]

The lack of an effective treatment has encouraged the exploration of lasers in the treatment of epistaxis.[25-30] Ben-Bassat,[25] using the CO_2 laser to cauterize nasal telangiectasias in 4 HHT patients, reported a reduction in the bleeding frequency after 1 to 10 laser treatments. Shapshay et al.[26,27] reported his experience with the Nd:YAG laser for photocoagulating nasal telangiectasias in 19 patients with varying degrees of severity of epistaxis, the latter classified according to the number of blood transfusions received. These authors reported that patients who had received either no or occasional transfusions responded well to laser treatment. By contrast, the ''end-stage'' group did not benefit from laser treatments.

Parkin used both argon and Nd:YAG lasers for treating epistaxis in HHT patients.[29] Nearly all patients reported improved results, but many required retreatments 4 to 6 months after the initial treatment. The KTP/532 nm laser has also been used to treat patients with epistaxis.[30] Although a marked decrease in the severity and frequency of epistaxis was reported, the followup period of this cohort was too short.

Although the CO_2, Nd:YAG, argon, and KTP lasers have all been used to treat HHT, the injury produced by each of these lasers has been a widespread, nonspecific thermal injury of the laser-exposed sites. Scar formation has been a severe and unwanted side effect resulting from these laser treatments. As is evident, scarring resulting from extensive laser treatment can ultimately prevent the use of these lasers from being an effective mode of treatment.

Therefore, because of the severity and chronicity of HHT, the ideal treatment should be one in which the damage remains localized to the abnormal blood vessels alone, and injury induced in normal, healthy adjacent tissues is kept to a minimum.

Angiokeratoma

There are several distinct types of angiokeratoma that share similar clinical and histologic features. Clinically, angiokeratomas present as asymptomatic hyperkeratotic erythematous papules (Fig. 12–9A). Histologically, there are varying degrees of hyperkeratosis and acanthosis, overlying widened dermal papillae, distended with dilated ectatic capillaries, lined by flat endothelial cells. The vessels may either appear empty or contain blood, which is occasionally thrombosed. There may also be ectatic vessels in the upper, mid, or lower dermis.

The rare angiokeratoma circumscriptum usually appears at birth and consists of coalesced papules, forming a plaque. In the Mibelli type, wartlike lesions appear, usually on the fingers and toes of adolescent girls, in association with chilblains. The Fordyce types is characterized by the appearance of solitary or multiple lesions on the scrotum (or vulva), increasing in number with maturation. Solitary or multiple papular angiokeratomas do not appear in childhood and are seen especially on the legs.

In the sex-linked inherited angiokeratoma corporis diffusum (Fabry's disease), the skin lesions appear around puberty, especially on the thighs, lower abdomen, and scrotum. The disorder arises from ceramide trihexosidase deficiency, leading to deposition of glycolipid in cutaneous and visceral blood vessels.

Because ectatic vessels are often present in the upper, mid, and lower dermis, the pulsed dye laser has effectively cleared these lesions at fluences of around 6.5 J/cm^2 (Fig. 12–9B). A higher fluence is required in this instance to enable the laser light to penetrate the hyperkeratosis overlying the ectatic dermal blood vessels.

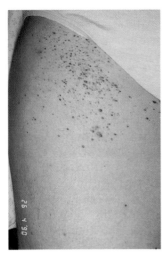 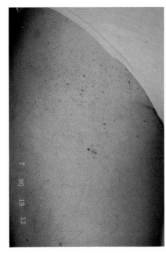

Fig. 12–9. *A.* Angiokeratoma on the posterior thigh. *B.* The same lesions following pulsed dye laser treatment.

A   B

Fig. 12–10. *A.* Pretreated pyogenic granuloma. *B.* The same lesion after multiple treatment using the pulsed dye laser. Note the absence of scarring of the treated site.

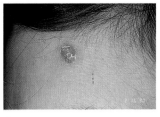
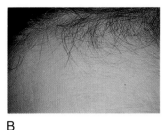

A   B

Pyogenic Granuloma

These tend to be single, raised, slightly pedunculated red lesions; they are often smooth, but they can superficially ulcerate and be crusted (Fig. 12–10A). Pyogenic granuloma bleed profusely when traumatized. Although most lesions are single, multiple lesions have been reported.[31]

Histopathologically, the capillary lumina, which can be small, cleftlike, or ectatic, are lined by prominent, proliferating endothelial cells.[31] The most significant histopathologic finding is the complete absence of Weibel-Palade bodies in the endothelial cells on electron microscopy.[32]

Problems associated with the treatment of these lesions include profuse bleeding during the procedure, enlargement instead of destruction of the tumor, and recurrence.

Because the lesions tend to extend deep into dermis, the most effective way of using the pulsed dye laser to treat them without inducing profuse bleeding is, first, to compress the lesion with a glass slide and then irradiate, using several pulses at fluences of between 7.5 and 8.0 J/cm^2. The glass slide is then removed and the lesion carefully irradiated with 7.0 to 8.0 J/cm^2, starting with multiple pulses at the base and gradually moving the beam to the "crown" of the lesion. If bleeding occurs at this stage, pressure and gel foam should be applied until hemostasis is achieved. A pressure dressing at this stage is also often very helpful.

Retreatments should be administered once every 3 to 4 weeks until the lesion decreases in size and eventually clears (Fig. 12–10B). Should the lesion proliferate rather than decrease in size with repeated laser treatments, those treatments should be discontinued and the lesion should be surgically removed. It is important, during discussions with the patient regarding treatment of the lesion, to stress that recurrence might occur and that the lesion might have to be surgically removed should laser treatments prove unsuccessful. The advantage of using the laser, it should be noted, is the absence of scar formation.

Angiofibroma (Adenoma Sebaceum)

Angiofibromas are commonly present in those with autosomal dominantly inherited tuberous sclerosis. The lesions usually develop before puberty and become more widespread thereafter. Clinically, they appear as discrete, firm, telangiectatic papules commonly seen on the cheeks, chin, and nasolabial folds (Fig. 12–11). Histologically, these papules are made up of dilated blood vessels, hyperplastic sebaceous glands, and immature follicles.

Angiofibroma is sometimes also used to designate such diverse entities as fibrous papules of the nose and pearly penile papules.

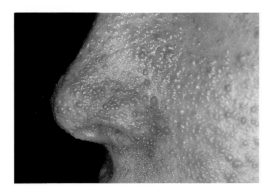

Fig. 12–11. Angiofibroma on the nose and malar regions.

Various techniques, including the laser, have been used to clear these lesions. Although some have been effective, the response in general has been temporary, and recurrence is almost always inevitable.

Blue Rubber Bleb Syndrome

Patients present with protuberant, dark blue, soft, some peduculated, compressible vascular tumors (Fig. 12–12), often present in the skin at birth and continuing to increase in size and number with maturation of the individual.[33] These lesions are not confined to the skin alone; they can also involve the gastrointestinal tract, causing chronic bleeding and anemia.[34] Lesions involving other viscera besides the gastrointestinal tract have also been reported to occur.[35]

In spite of their size, which can range from a few millimeters to several centimeters (Fig. 12–12), these cutaneous lesions have been "flattened" when exposed to the pulsed dye laser at fluences around 6.5 to 7.5 J/cm^2. Treatment of these lesions has not only made them cosmetically less conspicuous, but, more importantly, has reduced their size and thus decreased their susceptibility to trauma and bleeding. The latter can be very cumbersome.

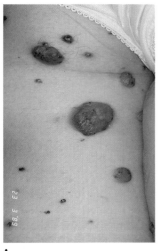

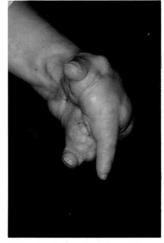

Fig. 12–12. *A.* Blue rubber bleb tumors on the posterior thigh. Note that the tumors can vary in size from a few millimeters to several centimeters. *B.* These tumors can involve other organs, such as the hand, besides the skin and gastrointestinal tract.

A   B

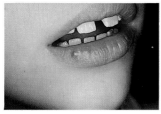
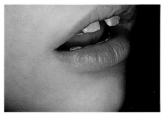

Fig. 12–13. Venous lake. *A*. Pre–pulsed dye laser treatment. *B*. Post-treatment.

A   B

Venous Lake

Venous lakes are dark blue, soft, raised lesions commonly found on the lips, ears, and face of elderly subjects (Fig. 12–13). Histopathologically, they are dilated veins or venules in the superficial papillary dermis; these vessels are lined by a single layer of flattened endothelial cells and a thin wall of fibrous tissue.[36]

The most effective way of treating the lesion using the pulsed dye laser is, first, to compress the lesion with a glass slide and irradiate it through the glass at around 6.5 to 7.0 J/cm^2. The glass slide is then removed and the lesion is exposed to several single pulses at 6.25 to 6.5 J/cm^2. Treated lesions will darken immediately, turning almost black within hours of laser exposure. The venous lake should be retreated once every 4 to 6 weeks until it disappears (Fig. 12–13).

Lymphangioma

Of the various lymphangiomas, lymphangioma circumscriptum is pertinent to this discussion. Blood-tinged, lymph-filled vesicles, usually grouped, are present on the skin in babies either at birth or at infancy. Histologically, dilated lymph capillaries are present in the dermal papillae lying beneath a hyperplastic epidermis.

The few cases which have presented for pulsed dye laser treatment have not been suitable for this treatment modality because the lesions have, in general, appeared clinically more "lymphatic" than vascular. This has meant that there has been insufficient hemoglobin (chromophore) within these lesions to absorb enough 577/585 nm laser energy to effectively destroy the abnormal tissue.

References

1. Goldman L, Blaney DJ, Kindel DJ, et al. Effect of the laser beam on the skin. J Invest Dermatol 40:121, 1963.
2. Apfelberg DB, Maser MR, Lash H. Extended clinical use of the argon laser for cutaneous lesions. Arch Dermatol 115:719, 1979.
3. Arndt KA. Argon laser therapy of small cutaneous vascular lesions. Arch Dermatol 118:220, 1982.
4. Hobby LW. Treatment of portwine stains and other cutaneous lesions. Contemp Surg 8:21, 1981.
5. Garden JM, Tan OT, Polla I, et al. The pulsed dye laser as a modality for treating cutaneous small blood vessel disease processes. Lasers Surg Med 6:259, 1986.
6. Goldman MP, Fitzpatrick RE. Pulsed dye laser treatment of leg telangiectasia: with and without simultaneous sclerotherapy. J Dermatol Surg Oncol 16:338, 1990.

7. Motemedi M, Welch AJ, Cheong WF, Chaffari S, Tan OT. Thermal lensing in biologic medium. IEEE J Quant Electron 24:693, 1988.
8. Tan OT, Motemedi M, Welch AJ, Kurban AK. Spotsize effects in guinea pig skin caused by pulsed irradiation. J Invest Dermatol 90:877, 1988.
9. Polla LL, Tan OT, Garden JM, Parrish JA. Tunable dye laser treatment of cutaneous vascular ectasia. Dermatologica 174:11, 1987.
10. Tan OT, Gilchrest BA. Selected cutaneous vascular lesions in the pediatric population. Pediatrics 82:652, 1988.
11. Goldman MP, Martin DE, Fitzpatrick RE, et al. Pulse dye laser treatment of telangiectasia with and without sub-therapeutic sclerotherapy: clinical and histologic examination in the rabbit ear vein model. J Am Acad Dermatol 23:23, 1990.
12. Tan OT, Morelli JG. Lasers in dermatology. Curr Probl Dermatol 1:1, 1989.
13. McGrae JD, Winkelman RK. Generalized essential telangiectasia: report of a clinical and histochemical study of 13 patients with acquired cutaneous lesions. JAMA 185:909, 1972.
14. Becker SW. Generalized telangiectasia: a clinical study with special consideration of etiology and pathology. Arch Dermatol 14:387, 1926.
15. Hutchinson J. A peculiar form of serpiginous infective naevoid disease. Arch Surg (Lindin) 1:Plate IX, 1889–1890.
16. Radcliffe-Crocker H. Diseases of the Skin. Philadelphia, Blakiston Press, 1893, p 646.
17. Shelley WB. Essential progressive telangiectasia. Successful treatment with tetracycline. JAMA 216:1343, 1971.
18. Wilson Jones E. Malignant vascular tumors. Clin Exp Dermatol 1:287, 1976.
19. Alessi E, Bertani E, Sala F. Acquired tufted angioma. Am J Dermatopathol 8:426, 1986.
20. Wilson Jones E, Orkin M. Tufted angioma (angioblastoma). J Am Acad Dermatol 20:214, 1989.
21. Padilla RS, Orkin M, Rosai R, Acquired "tufted" angioma (progressive capillary hemangioma). Am J Dermatopathol 9:292, 1987.
22. Hashimoto K, Pritzker MS. Hereditary hemorrhagic telangiectasia, an electron microscopic study. Oral Surg 34:751, 1972.
23. McCabe WP, Kelly AP Jr. Management of epistaxis in Osler-Weber-Rendu disease: recurrence of telangiectasias with a nasal skin graft. Plast Reconstr Surg 50:114, 1972.
24. Richtsmeier W, Weaver G, Streck W, et al. Estrogen and progesterone receptors in hereditary hemorrhagic telangiectasia. Otolaryngol Head Neck Surg 92:564, 1984.
25. Ben-Bassat M, Kaplan I, Levy R. Treatment of hereditary hemorrhagic telangiectasia of the nasal mucosa with the carbon dioxide laser. Br J Plast Surg 31:157, 1978.
26. Shapshay SM, Oliver P. Treatment of hereditary hemorrhagic telangiectasia by Nd:YAG laser photocoagulation. Laryngoscope 94:1554, 1984.
27. Kluger PB, Shapshay SM. Neodymium-YAG laser intranasal photocoagulation in hereditary hemorrhagic telangiectasia: an update report. Laryngoscope 97:1397, 1987.
28. Parkin JL, Dixon JA. Laser photocoagulation in hereditary hemorrhagic telangiectasia. Otolaryngol Head Neck Surg 89:204, 1981.
29. Parkin JL, Dixon JA. Argon laser treatment of head and neck vascular lesions. Otolaryngol Head Neck Surg 93:211, 1985.
30. Levine HL. Endoscopy and the KTP/532 laser for nasal sinus disease. Ann Otol Rhinol Laryngol 98:46, 1989.
31. Coskey RJ, Mehregan AH. Granuloma pyogenicum with multiple satellite recurrences. Arch Dermatol 96:71, 1967.
32. Davis MG, Barton SP, Atai F, et al. The abnormal dermis in pyogenic granuloma. J Am Acad Dermatol 2:132, 1980.
33. Bean WB. Vascular Spiders and Related Lesions of the Skin. Springfield IL, Charles C Thomas, 1958, pp 178–185.
34. Fretzin DF, Potter B. Blue rubber bleb nevus. Arch Intern Med 116:924, 1965.
35. Rice JS, Fischer DS. Blue rubber-bleb nevus syndrome. Arch Dermatol 86:503, 1962.
36. Bean WB, Walsh JR. Venous lakes. Arch Dermatol 74:459, 1956.

Chapter 13　Leg Veins: Pathogenesis, Sclerotherapy, and Lasers

Mitchel P. Goldman

Unsightly or symptomatic venulectases and/or telangiectasias on the legs occur in 29 to 41% of women and 6 to 15% of men in the United States.[1] The family history of varicose or telangiectatic leg veins ranges from 43[2] to 90%.[3] Approximately one-third of patients first note the development of these veins during pregnancy. Between 20 and 30% of patients develop these veins prior to pregnancy, with 18% of women noting the onset while ingesting progestational agents. The development of "spider leg veins," therefore, is probably a partially sex-linked, autosomal dominant condition with incomplete penetrance and variable expressivity.

Even though up to 53% of patients have associated symptoms from these veins, the most common reason patients seek treatment is cosmetic.[4] Therefore, any treatment that is effective should be relatively free of adverse sequelae. Unfortunately, all forms of treatment to date have negative side effects.[5]

The most common method for treating leg telangiectasia is sclerotherapy. Up to 30% of patients treated with sclerotherapy will develop postsclerosis pigmentation[6] and telangiectatic matting.[7] Postsclerosis hyperpigmentation is caused by the extravasation of erythrocytes through sclerotherapy-damaged or destroyed vessels.[6] This is more likely to occur if sclerosing agents of excessive strength are utilized, but may occur even with optimal treatment.[6,8] Telangiectatic matting is thought to be related to the use of excessively strong sclerosing agents with the development of "excessive" perivascular inflammation[5,9] or "excessive" thrombus formation.[9]

Various forms of laser have been utilized in an effort to enhance clinical efficacy and minimize the adverse sequelae from sclerotherapy. Unfortunately, most forms of laser treatment have also been associated with a number of adverse sequelae far in excess of those associated with sclerotherapy. This chapter reviews the present literature on laser treatment of leg telangiectasia and presents a rational treatment plan for its use as part of the overall treatment strategy.

Pathophysiology of Leg Telangiectasia

Telangiectasias may be classified into four types (linear, arborizing, spider, and papular) based on clinical appearance.[10] Two common patterns of telangiectasia on the legs of women, besides red or blue streaks, are the parallel linear pattern, especially found on the medial thigh (Fig. 13–1), and the arborizing or radiating cartwheel pattern, especially seen on the lateral thigh (Fig. 13–2).[11] These two subsets of telangiectasia seem to run in families and may form anastomosing complexes that may be as large as 15 cm in diameter. They may appear with or without "feeding" reticular veins.

Telangiectasias which originate from arterioles on the arterial side of a capillary loop tend to be small, bright red, and do not protrude above the skin surface. Telangiectasias which originate from venules on the venous side of a capillary loop, on the other hand, are blue, wider, and often protrude above the skin surface. Sometimes telangiectasias, especially those arising at the capillary loop, are at first red, but with time become blue probably because of increasing hydrostatic pressure and back-flow from the venous side.[12]

Varicose veins most likely lead to the development of telangiectasia either through associated venous hypertension with resulting angiogenesis or vascular dilatation[12] and/or through an associated increased distensibility of the telangiectatic vein wall. Although telangiectasias associated with varicose veins may appear at first as erythematous streaks, with time they turn blue. Often they are directly associated with underlying varicose veins so that the

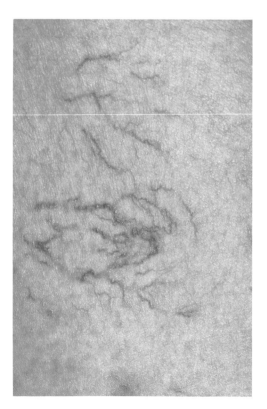

Fig. 13–1. Typical appearance of telangiectasia located on the medial thigh of a 54-year-old woman. Note the feeding reticular vein proximal to the telangiectasia.

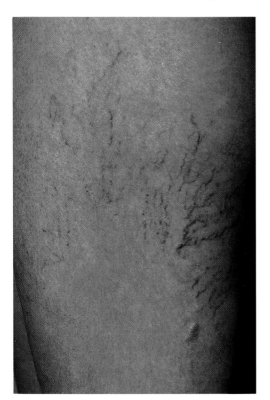

Fig. 13–2. Common appearance of cartwheel or radiating telangiectasia pattern on the lateral thigh of a 42-year-old woman. Note the feeding blue reticular vein at the distal aspect of the telangiectatic pattern.

distinction between telangiectasias and varicose veins becomes blurred.[12] Tretbar demonstrated that telangiectasias are associated with underlying reticular veins.[13] These veins were separate from any truncal varicosities that might have been present. All blue reticular veins demonstrated reflux that did not appear to originate from the long or short saphenous veins. Fifty percent of patients with blue reticular veins demonstrated reflux from incompetent calf-perforating veins. In this scenario, treatment of the feeding varicosity results in treatment of the distal telangiectasia. Finally, when no apparent connection exists between deep collecting or reticular vessels, the telangiectasia may arise from a terminal arteriole or arteriovenous anastomosis.[14]

Telangiectasia may be associated with underlying venous disease even when there are no clinical abnormalities. Twenty-three percent of patients without clinically apparent varicose veins examined with duplex imaging and venous Doppler demonstrated incompetence of the superficial venous system.[15] In addition, 1.2% had incompetence of a perforator vein. Nineteen patients with one clinically abnormal leg and one clinically normal leg were also evaluated. Interestingly, 37% of clinically normal legs demonstrated incompetence of the superficial system. The abnormal leg in this group had a 74% incidence of incompetence of the superficial system, with 21% having saphenofemoral incompetence. This study demonstrates the need for both a clinical and noninvasive diagnostic work-up in patients who present with telangiectatic leg veins and also reinforces the view that "spider" leg veins arise from underlying varicose veins via venous hypertension.

A proposed mechanism for the development of leg telangiectasia associated with underlying venous disease is that pre-existing vascular anastomotic channels open in response to venous stasis.[16] The resulting capillary hypertension leads to opening and dilatation of normally closed vessels. Alternatively, relative anoxia as a result of reversed venous flow leads to angiogenesis.[14]

The hormonal influence in the development of telangiectasia is well known. Perhaps the most common physiologic condition which leads to the development of telangiectasia is pregnancy. Almost 70% of women develop telangiectasias during pregnancy, the majority of which disappear between 3 and 6 weeks post partum.[12] Pregnant women often develop telangiectasias on the legs within a few weeks of conception, even before the uterus has enlarged to compress venous return to the pelvis.[17,18] In addition, pregnant women and those taking the birth control pill have been shown to have an increase in the distensibility of vein walls.[19] This increase in distensibility has also been noted to fluctuate with the normal menstrual cycle.[20] It was found that leg volume was greatest just before ovulation and during menses. Thus, some hormonal influence is involved in the development of varicose veins and their associated telangiectasias in women. Finally, there is an apparent association of estrogen excess states with the development of telangiectatic matting following sclerotherapy of spider leg veins. Twenty-nine percent of women who developed ''new'' telangiectasia were taking systemic estrogens or became pregnant, as compared to 19% of patients on hormones who did not develop telangiectatic matting.[21]

Histology of Leg Telangiectasia

The venules in the upper and mid dermis usually run in a horizontal orientation. The diameter of the postcapillary venule ranges from 12 to 35 μm.[22] Collecting venules range from 40 to 60 μm in the upper and mid dermis and enlarge to 100 to 400 μm in diameter in the deeper tissues.[23] One-way valves are found at the subcutis (dermis)–adipose junction on the venous side of the circulation.[24] Valves are usually found in the area of anastomosis of small to large venules and also within larger venules unassociated with branching points. The free edges of the valves are always directed from the smaller to larger vessel so blood flows towards the deeper venous system (Fig. 13–3).

Histologic examination of simple telangiectasias demonstrates dilated blood channels in a normal dermal stroma with a single endothelial cell lining,

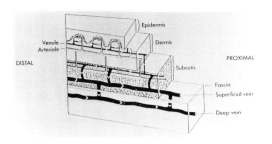

Fig. 13–3. Schematic diagram of the cutaneous and subcutaneous vascular plexus. (Reproduced with permission from: Goldman MP. Sclerotherapy Treatment of Varicose and Telangiectatic Leg Veins. St. Louis, Mosby-Year Book, Inc., 1991.)

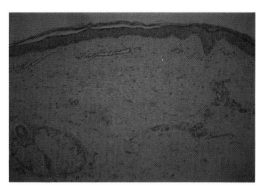 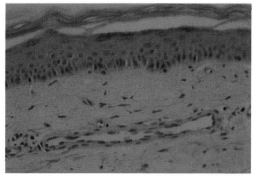

Fig. 13–4. Typical location and diameter of a linear telangiectasia on the thigh of a 45-year-old woman (hematoxylin-eosin; *A,* ×100; *B,* ×400).

limited muscularis, and adventitia[5] (Fig. 13–4). Blue-to-red arborizing telangiectasias of the lower extremities are probably dilated venules, possibly with intimate and direct connections to underlying larger veins from which they are direct tributaries.[12,25,26] Most leg telangiectasias measure between 26 and 225 μm in diameter.[26] Electron microscopic examination of "sunburst" varicosities of the leg has demonstrated that these vessels are widened cutaneous veins.[27] They are found 175 to 382 μm below the stratum granulosum. The thickened vessel walls are composed of endothelial cells covered with collagen and muscle fibers. Elastic fibers are also present. Electron microscopy reveals an intercellular collagenous dysplasia, lattice collagen, and some matrix vesicles. These findings suggest that telangiectatic leg veins, like varicose veins, have an alteration of collagen metabolism of their walls. Therefore, like varicose veins, these veins are dysplastic. Alternatively, arteriovenous anastomoses may result in the pathogenesis of telangiectasias. Arteriovenous anastamoses have also been demonstrated in 1 of 26 biopsy specimens of leg telangiectasia.[26]

Unlike leg telangiectasia, nevus flammeus (port-wine stain) under histologic examination shows a collection of thin-walled capillary and cavernous vessels arranged in a loose fashion throughout the superficial and deep dermis. These vessels represent dilatations of the postcapillary venules of the superficial dermis with a mean vessel depth of 0.46 mm.[28] They are much smaller than leg telangiectasia, usually measuring 10 to 40 μm in diameter.[29] Rarely, cavernous hemangiomas arising from arteriovenous malformations may occur within the lesions.[30] There may also be evidence of neovascularization or other vascular malformation.[28] Therefore, the vasculature of nevus flammeus is different from leg telangiectasia. This may explain the lack of efficacy reported by many physicians who treat leg telangiectasia with the same laser parameters as port-wine hemangioma.

Sclerotherapy Treatment of Leg Telangiectasias

Treatment of varicose veins by first closing off the high pressure reflux points with a small volume of sclerosant followed by sclerotherapy of remaining abnormal vessels forms the basis for rational compression

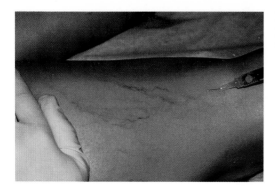

Fig. 13–5. Correct placement of first injection into leg telangiectasia arising from a "feeding" reticular vein.

sclerotherapy of varicose veins.[8] Since, in the vast majority of cases, spider veins are in direct connection to underlying varicose veins either directly or through tributaries, as with varicose veins, treatment should first be directed to "plugging" the leaking high-pressure outflow at its point of origin. An appropriate analogy is to think of the spider veins as the fingers and the feeding varicose vein as the arm. Treatment should first be directed to the feeding "arm" and then, only if necessary, directly to the spider "fingers" (Fig. 13–5). There are a number of advantages to this systematic approach to sclerotherapy. When performed in this manner, the spider veins often disappear without their direct treatment, thus limiting the number of injections into the patient. The larger feeding vein is both easier to cannulate and less likely to rupture with injection of the sclerosant, thus minimizing the extent of extravasated RBCs and sclerosant. Theoretically, this method should minimize treatment complications.

A complete discussion of sclerotherapy treatment is beyond the scope of this chapter. The reader is referred to a recent textbook on this subject.[8] The essential point is that all leg telangiectasia which can be cannulated with a 30-gauge needle should be treated before considering laser surgery. Treatment should proceed from the largest to the smallest vessel. Only those vessels which do not respond to sclerotherapy or those vessels which are too small to be injected should be considered for laser treatment. By adhering to these principles, physicians will provide their patients with cost-effective, efficient, and logical care.

Laser Treatment of Leg Telangiectasias

Carbon Dioxide

The carbon dioxide (CO_2) laser has been used for the obliteration of venules and telangiectatic vessels.[11,31–33] The CO_2 laser emits light energy at 10,600 nm in the infrared portion of the electromagnetic spectrum, thereby producing nonspecific thermal vaporization of all tissue structures in its path. The rationale for using the CO_2 laser in the treatment of telangiectasias is to produce precise vaporization without significant damage to tissue structures adjacent to the penetrating laser beam. However, the skin surface, as well as the dermis overlying the blood vessel, is destroyed. Carbon dioxide laser penetration of vessels has also been reported to cause occasional brisk bleeding from the vessel that required pressure bandages for 48 hours.[32] Pain during treatment is moderate to severe, but of short duration. All reported studies demonstrate unsatisfactory cosmetic results. Treated areas show multiple hypopigmented punctate scars with either minimal resolution of the treated vessel or neovascularization adjacent to the treatment site. Because of this nonselective action, the CO_2 laser is of no advantage over the electrodesiccation needle and has not been successfully utilized in treating leg telangiectasia.

Neodymium:YAG

The neodymium:YAG (Nd:YAG) laser at 1060 nm has also been used to treat leg telangiectasias.[32] The average depth of penetration in human skin is 0.75 mm, and reduction to 10% of the incident power occurs at a depth of 3.7 mm.[34] Thus, this laser is well-suited to treat blood vessels within the mid dermis. However, the wavelength is absorbed by water, and to a certain degree by melanin and hemoglobin. Therefore, as with the CO_2 laser, tissue damage is relatively nonspecific. Apfelberg[32] treated leg telangiectasias with the Nd:YAG laser equipped with a 1.5 mm sapphire contact probe. Treatment complications included linear hypopigmentation, depressions overlying the skin of the treated vessel, and the need to retreat the vessels at 6-week intervals. In addition, the cost is high because the disposable sapphire tips are expensive. In summary, as reported with the CO_2 laser, this modality produces unsatisfactory cosmetic results and has yet to be found useful in treating leg telangiectasias.

Argon

The argon laser is theoretically better suited for treating telangiectasias. The blue-green light emits 80% of its energy at 488/514 nm. Since oxygenated hemoglobin located in the superficial dermal ectatic blood vessels has absorption peaks at 418, 542, and 577 nm, selective absorption of the argon laser spectrum occurs. Argon laser light passes through the skin surface into the upper reticular dermis for a distance of about 1 mm in caucasian skin.[35] Unfortunately, argon laser light is not entirely hemoglobin-specific. The epidermis absorbs the 488/514 nm wavelengths about half as strongly as blood and is therefore nontransparent.[36] Epidermal melanin also absorbs a variable portion of argon laser light. This may result in hypopigmentation of the treated areas. Thus, the specificity of argon laser-induced damage appears to be much less than originally hypothesized.

In addition to the relative nonspecificity of the argon laser wavelength for oxygenated hemoglobin, presently available argon lasers deliver energy exposures with pulse durations only as short as 50 msec. This minimal exposure still allows time for extensive radial diffusion and dissipation of heat generated in the treated blood vessels, thereby resulting in a relatively nonselective thermal destruction.[37] In practice, for the argon laser to produce clinically effective results, pulses are delivered until tissue whitening occurs.[38] This whitening represents nonspecific thermal damage to the epidermis and dermis and not simply blanching of the vascular bed. In fact, there appears to be no clinical difference between continuous-wave therapy and 50 msec pulse therapy.[38] Thus, there is a risk of hypertrophic or atrophic scarring secondary to nonspecific epidermal and upper dermal necrosis and subsequent fibrosis. This is noted clinically by epidermal sloughing postoperatively, followed by crusting and gradual re-epithelialization over 1 to 2 weeks.[39] Typically, pitted, hypertrophic, and depressed scars have been observed.[40–48] Hyper- or hypopigmentation has been reported in 32 to 44% of patients.[40,49,50]

Telangiectasias or superficial varicosities of the lower extremities are much less responsive to laser treatment. Treated areas in this location usually appear purple or depressed, often leaving a worse cosmetic appearance than the untreated condition.[51,52] In a report of 38 patients treated by Apfelberg et al.,[53] 49% had either poor or no results from treatment; only 16% had excellent or good results. In addition, almost half of the patients had hemosiderin bruising. In another series, Dixon et al.[54] noted significant improvement in only 49% of patients. They speculated that after initial improvement, incomplete thrombosis, recanalization, or new vein formation produced reappearance of the vessels after 6 to 12 months.

In an effort to enhance therapeutic success with sclerotherapy, the argon laser has been used to interrupt the flow of blood in the telangiectasia every 2 to 3 cm prior to injection of the sclerosing agent.[55] Eleven of 16 patients completed treatment. Two patients developed punctate depigmented scars, and hyperpigmentation appeared in 3 additional patients. However, 93.7% of patients had ''satisfactory'' results. Thus, at the present time, while argon-laser therapy appears to be a satisfactory method for treating selected facial telangiectasias, it is much less effective in treating leg telangiectasias.

Pulsed Dye Laser (PDL), 585 nm

A new pulsed dye laser system (Candela Model SPTL-1 Pulsed Dye Laser) has been reported to be highly efficacious in the treatment of cutaneous vascular lesions. The depth of vascular damage is estimated to be 1.2 mm at 585 nm while maintaining the same degree of vascular selectivity as that previously described for 577 nm irradiation.[56] Therefore, the PDL can treat the typical depth of leg telangiectasia.

To ensure highly specific vessel damage the laser energy must also be delivered in a period of time which is less than that required for the cooling of the target vessel, i.e., less than the thermal relaxation time. For superficial cutaneous blood vessels, thermal relaxation times average 1.2 msec.[57] Tan et. al.,[59] using 300 μsec pulses, demonstrated specific intravascular damage with destruction of endothelial cells.

Studies utilizing a 577 nm dye laser with a 300 μsec pulse demonstrate minimal perivascular or epidermal damage[58] and no evidence of scarring after treatment.[59] However, although very effective for facial port-wine hemangiomas, telangiectasias, spider ectasia, and capillary hemangiomas, telangiectasias over the lower extremities have not responded as well, with less lightening and more post-therapy hyperpigmentation.[60] This may result from the larger diameter of the leg telangiectasia compared to the dermal vessels in nevus flammeus (see histology section), or from the failure to recognize the importance of high-pressure vascular flow from feeding reticular and varicose veins.

Polla et al.[61] treated 35 superficial leg telangiectasias with the PDL. The exact laser parameters were not given, except that vessels were treated an average of 2.1 times with a maximum of 4 separate treatments. These vessels were described as being either red-purple and raised or blue and flat. No mention was made regarding the association of reticular or varicose veins. No mention was made of the vessel diameter. Fifteen percent of treated vessels had greater than 75% clearing, with 73% of treated areas showing little response to treatment. The only lesions which responded at all were the tiny red-pink telangiectasias. Almost 50% of treated patients developed a persistent hypo- or hyperpigmentation of treated sites.

As illustrated in the above-mentioned study, it is difficult to compare the clinical and experimental studies of laser treatment of leg telangiectasia with that of port-wine stain. Laser studies on the treatment of leg telangiectasias typically do not report the diameter, location, or type of vessel treated. In addition, no mention is made of ''feeding'' varicosities or of postlaser compression. Therefore, we systematically examined the clinical effects of various powers of the PDL in specific leg telangiectasias. We chose for examination red telangiectasia less than 0.2 mm in diameter and vessels arising as a function of telangiectatic matting since these vessels are the most difficult to treat with standard sclerotherapy techniques.

Simultaneous Laser/Sclerotherapy Treatment

The use of subtherapeutic concentrations of sclerosing solutions in combination with highly specific laser-induced endothelial damage may result in an enhanced efficacy with laser treatment of larger blood vessels. The combination pulsed dye laser/sclerotherapy technique (PDL/SCL) and pulsed dye laser (PDL) alone are hypothesized to result in a decreased incidence of extravasation of erythrocytes and decreased perivascular inflammation. In addition, PDL with its resulting thermal endothelial damage should inhibit angiogenesis.[62] Thus, PDL and PDL/SCL may result in a decreased incidence of adverse sequelae (postsclerotherapy hyperpigmentation and telangiectatic matting).

The PDL produces vascular injury in a histologic pattern that is different from that produced by sclerotherapy. In a previous study on an identical animal model,[63] approximately 50% of vessels treated with an effective concentration of sclerosant demonstrated extravasated RBCs (unpublished observations). In the rabbit ear vein model, extravasated RBCs were apparent in 30% of vessels treated with the PDL alone or in combination with sclerotherapy. Thus, PDL and/or PDL/SCL may produce less post-therapy pigmentation because of a decreased incidence of extravasated RBCs.

The cause of telangiectatic matting is unknown but has been thought to be related either to angiogenesis[64] or a dilatation of existing subclinical blood vessels by promoting collateral flow through arteriovenous anastomoses.[65] One or both of these mechanisms may occur. Obstruction of outflow from a vessel (which is the end result of successful sclerotherapy) is one of the most important factors contributing to angiogenesis.[66] In addition, endothelial damage leads to the release of histamine and other mast-cell factors, promoting both the dilatation of existing blood vessels and angiogenesis.[67,68] Thus, sclerotherapy by its very mechanism of action provides the mechanisms for new blood-vessel formation to occur. Indeed, it is remarkable that one does not see an increased incidence of postsclerosis telangiectatic matting with sclerotherapy treatment.

Telangiectatic matting has not been reported to be a side effect from argon, PDL, and/or dye laser treatment of any vascular disorders. This may be because the production of intravascular fibrin occurs during laser treatment.[69–71] This is believed to occur through thermal alteration of fibrin complexes. Fibrin deposition has been demonstrated to promote angiogenesis.[72] Interestingly, sclerotherapy-induced vascular injury has not been associated with the appearance of fibrin strands (unpublished observations). Therefore, either factors other than those associated with the absence of fibrin deposition or the intravascular consumption of fibrin-promoting factors must be limiting angiogenesis in PDL treatment of cutaneous vascular disease.

Another possible mechanism for the decrease in telangiectatic matting in laser-treated blood vessels may be a decrease in perivascular inflammation. PDL and PDL/SCL result in a relative decrease in perivascular inflammation compared to vessels treated with sclerotherapy alone.[70] Multiple factors associated with inflammation have been demonstrated to promote both a dilatation of existing blood vessels and angiogenesis.[72] Thus, a relative decrease in perivascular inflammation may also be responsible for the absence of telangiectatic matting in laser-treated areas.

Evaluation of PDL Treatment of Leg Telangiectasia

The above-mentioned theoretic advantages and methods for treating leg telangiectasia with the PDL or PDL/SCL were examined by Goldman and Fitzpatrick.[73] Thirty female patients with an average age of 38 years (range 20–67) who presented for treatment of telangiectatic leg veins were treated (Fig. 13–6). The telangiectatic patches that measured less than 0.2 mm in diameter were red in color. Thirteen of 101 telangiectatic patches were noted to have an associated reticular feeding vein between 2 and 3 mm in diameter that was not treated. Seven patients with 25 patches of telangiectatic matting after previous sclerotherapy were also treated.

PDL 5 mm diameter spots were overlapped slightly, with every effort made to treat the entire vessel. After treatment, a Kwik Kold chemical ice pack was applied to the treated area until the laser-induced sensation of heat resolved (5–15 minutes). Thirty-nine telangiectatic patches, chosen randomly, were treated with laser energies between 7.0 and 8.0 J/cm^2 and compressed with a rubber "E" compression pad fixed in place with Microfoam 100 mm tape. A class II 30 to 40 mm Hg graduated compression stocking was then continuously worn over this dressing for approximately 72 hours.

As hypothesized, telangiectatic matting and persistent pigmentation did not occur with PDL treatment. All patients with post–PDL-induced hyperpigmentation completely resolved within 4 months. There were no episodes of cutaneous ulceration, thrombophlebitis, or other complications. However, recently we have seen hypopigmentation develop on the anterior thigh in a 27-year-old woman with very tan skin treated for telangiectatic matting with

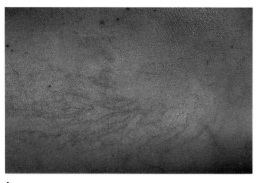

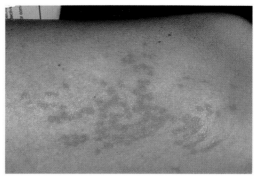

A

B

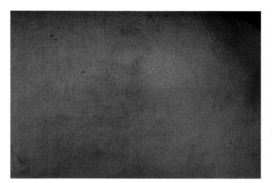

C

Fig. 13–6. PDL treatment of telangiectasia 0.2 mm in diameter on the left medial thigh of a 33-year-old woman. *A.* Before treatment. *B.* Immediately after treatment with the PDL at 7.0 J/cm^2, 125 5 mm laser impacts. *C.* Three months post-treatment with 100% resolution of telangiectasia. Slight light-brown hyperpigmentation is present and resolved within 4 weeks. (Reproduced with permission from: Goldman MP. Sclerotherapy Treatment of Varicose and Telangiectatic Leg Veins. St. Louis, Mosby-Year Book, Inc., 1991.)

the PDL alone at 7.25 J/cm^2. The laser impact sites remained hypopigmented for 6 months.

With PDL treatment, the most effective laser energy appears to be between 7.0 and 8.0 J/cm^2. At these laser parameters between 48 and 67% of telangiectatic patches were totally faded within 4 months. When telangiectatic patches with untreated feeding reticular veins are excluded, an average of 68% of telangiectatic patches totally faded.

There appeared to be no difference in the response to PDL in telangiectatic matting vessels. In 7 patients with 25 sites treated, 72% of the treated sites completely faded at laser energies between 6.5 and 7.5 J/cm^2. Telangiectatic matting vessels did not respond to treatment in only 1 patient with 4 areas of matting. Less than 90% resolution occurred in 16% of treated areas.

The reason for the greater efficacy of treatment in our report compared to others[60,61] may reflect the rigid criteria by which patients were selected for treatment. Our patients who responded well to treatment had red telangiectasia less than 0.2 mm in diameter without associated feeding reticular veins.

Many physicians have found that vessel location may affect treatment outcome, with vessels on the medial thigh being the most difficult to completely resolve. With the PDL, however, vessel location appears to be unrelated to treatment outcome if telangiectatic patches with untreated feeding reticular veins are excluded. In addition, there appeared to be no obvious difference in treatment efficacy between telangiectatic patches that were treated with compression and those that were not.

Evaluation of PDL/SCL Treatment of Leg Telangiectasia

Twenty-seven patients had either bilaterally symmetric telangiectatic patches or a large "starburst" telangiectatic flair that could be divided into two separate treatment sites. These 27 patients were treated at one site either with the PDL alone as described above, or with laser energies 1 to 2 J/cm^2 less than those utilized with PDL alone immediately before injection of the telangiectasia with Polidocanol, 0.25, 0.5, or 0.75% with a volume of 0.1 to 0.25 ml per injection site.[71]

Forty-four percent of treated areas completely resolved. There appeared to be little difference in efficacy and adverse sequelae with concentrations of Polidocanol from 0.25 to 0.75%. There did appear to be an increased efficacy of treatment with laser energies of 7.5 to 7.75 J/cm^2. As with PDL alone, treatment site did not appear to significantly affect treatment outcome except for an increased incidence of complications in the ankle and knee area.

The most significant difference between PDL alone and PDL/SCL was the incidence of complications to treatment. With combination PDL/SCL treatment, post-treatment ulceration and telangiectatic matting occurred in 11% of patient treatment areas. Six of 23 nonulcerated treatment sites developed persistent pigmentation beyond 1 year. Two of 27 sites developed telangiectatic matting that lasted over 1 year. Four of 27 treatment sites developed superficial ulceration; in these ulcerated patients, laser energies were equal to or greater than 6.5 J/cm^2, and Polidocanol concentration was equal to or greater than 0.5%.

In conclusion, the Candela SPTL-1 Pulsed Dye Laser at 585 nm is an effective modality for treatment of red leg telangiectasia less than or equal to 0.2 mm in diameter. PDL treatment is efficacious for both essential telangiectasia and vessels arising through the phenomenon of telangiectatic matting. This form of treatment alone has a remarkably low incidence of adverse sequelae. The optimal clinically useful laser energy with the Candela SPTL-1 laser in the treatment of red, 0.2 mm diameter telangiectatic mats is between 7.0 and 8.0 J/cm^2. Treatment is most efficacious if all vessels larger than 0.2 mm in diameter, especially varicose and reticular feeding veins, are treated first. Treatment results are not affected by vessel location. And, post-treatment compression of the vessels appears unnecessary with this type of vessel. Combination PDL/SCL treatment appears to offer no advantage to sclerotherapy treatment alone and appears to have a significant degree of complications when treatment is limited to red telangiectasia less than 0.2 mm in diameter (Table 13–1).

There is theoretic evidence to suggest that PDL/SCL treatment may be more efficacious than either PDL or sclerotherapy alone in the rabbit ear vein model.[70] Alone, in the rabbit ear vein model, the PDL was only effective in establishing a histologic and clinical resolution of the vessel when an energy of 10.0 J/cm^2 was utilized. In combination with immediate injection of the sclerosant (PDL/SCL), a significant degree of clinical and histologic resolution of the vessel occurred with all tested laser energies (8.0 to 10.0 J/cm^2). Pilot studies utilizing either sclerotherapy with Polidocanol 0.25% or treated with PDL laser energies of 6.0 and 7.0 J/cm^2 alone demonstrated no endothelial damage in vessels. However, the combination of PDL/SCL treated vessels at 6.0 and 7.0 J/cm^2 did demonstrate endothelial vacuolization. Thus, it is possible that PDL energies less than 5.0 J/cm^2 may be successfully

Table 13–1. Results Using Pulsed Dye Laser/Sclerotherapy vs. Pulsed Dye Laser Alone in the Treatment of Leg Telangiectasia

	Number of Patients	*No Change*	*Change %*	*Total fade*	*Ulcer/Matting*
PDL	91	19%	25%	56%	0%
PDL*	78	15%	20%	65%	9%
PDL/SCL	27	11%	33%	44%	11%

* = less patients with feeding reticular veins.

(Reproduced with permission from: Goldman MP, Fitzpatrick RE. Pulsed-dye laser treatment of leg telangiectasia: with and without simultaneous sclerotherapy. J Dermatol Surg Oncol 16:338, 1990.)

combined with sclerotherapy in human leg veins to provide effective therapy. In addition, a relative decrease in the extent of extravasated red blood cells and perivascular inflammation was noted in both PDL and PDL/SCL. Future studies on the use of PDL/SCL treatment of larger diameter blood vessels appear necessary.

References

1. Engel A, Johnson ML, Haynes SG. Health effects of sunlight exposure in the United States: results from the first national health and nutrition examination survey, 1971–1974. Arch Dermatol 124:72, 1988.
2. Sadick NS. Treatment of varicose and telangiectatic leg veins with hypertonic saline: a comparative study of heparin and saline. J Dermatol Surg Oncol 16:24, 1990.
3. Duffy DM. Small vessel sclerotherapy: an overview. *In* Advances in Dermatology. Vol 3. Edited by Callen, Dahl, Golitz, et al. Chicago, Year Book Medical Publishers Inc., 1988, pp 221–242.
4. Weiss RA, Weiss MA. Resolution of pain associated with varicose and telangiectatic leg veins after compression sclerotherapy. J Dermatol Surg Oncol 16:333, 1990.
5. Goldman MP, Bennett RG. Treatment of telangiectasia: a review. J Am Acad Dermatol 17:167, 1987.
6. Goldman MP, Kaplan RP, Duffy DM. Postsclerotherapy hyperpigmentation: a histologic evaluation. J Dermatol Surg Oncol 13:547, 1987.
7. Duffy DM. Small vessel sclerotherapy: an overview. *In* Advances in Dermatology. Vol 3. Edited by Callen, Dahl, Golitz, et al. Chicago, Year Book Medical Publishers Inc., 1988, pp 221–242.
8. Goldman MP. Sclerotherapy Treatment of Varicose and Telangiectatic Leg Veins. St. Louis, Mosby-Year Book, Inc., 1991.
9. Ouvry PA, Davy A. The sclerotherapy of telangiectasia. Phlebologie 35:349, 1982.
10. Redisch W, Pelzer RH. Localized vascular dilatations of the human skin: capillary microscopy and related studies. Am Heart J 37:106, 1949.
11. Kaplan I, Peled I. The carbon dioxide laser in the treatment of superficial telangiectasias. Br J Plast Surg 28:214, 1975.
12. Bean WB. Vascular Spiders and Related Lesions of the Skin. Springfield IL, Charles C. Thomas Publisher, 1958.
13. Tretbar LL. The origin of reflux in incompetent blue reticular/telangiectasia veins. *In* Phlebologie '89. Edited by Davy A, Stemmer R. Paris, John Libby Eurotext Ltd., 1989, pp 95–96.
14. Merelen JF. Telangiectasies rouges, telangiectasies bleues. Phlebologie 23:167, 1970.
15. Thibault P, Bray A. Cosmetic leg veins: evaluation using duplex venous imaging. J Dermatol Surg Oncol 16:612, 1990.
16. Curri GB, Lo Brutto ME. Influenza dei mucopolisaccaridi e dei loro costituenti sulla neoformazione vascolare. Rev Pat Clin Sper 8:379, 1967.
17. Miller SS. Investigation and management of varicose veins. Ann R Coll Surg Engl 55:245, 1974.
18. Mullane DJ. Varicose veins of pregnancy. Am J Obstet Gynecol 63:620, 1952.

19. Goodrich SM, Wood JE. Peripheral venous distensibility and velocity of venous blood flow during pregnancy or during oral contraceptive therapy. Am J Obstet Gynecol 90:740, 1964.

20. Keates JS, Fitzgerald DE. An interim report on lower limb volume and blood flow changes during a normal menstrual cycle. 5th Eur Conf Microcirculation, Gothenburg. Bibl Anat 10:189, 1968.

21. Davis LT, Duffy DM. Determination of incidence and risk factors for post-sclerotherapy telangiectatic matting of the lower extremity: a retrospective analysis. J Dermatol Surg Oncol 16:327, 1990.

22. Braverman IM. Ultrastructure and organization of the cutaneous microvasculature in normal and pathologic states. J Invest Dermatol 93:2S, 1989.

23. Miami A, Rubertsi U. Collecting venules. Minerva Cardioangiol 41:541, 1958.

24. Braverman IM, Keh-Yen A. Ultrastructure of the human dermal microcirculation. IV. Valve-containing collecting veins at the dermal-subcutaneous junction. J Invest Dermatol 81:438, 1983.

25. Bodian EL. Sclerotherapy. Semin Dermatol 6:238, 1987.

26. Faria JL de, Moraes IN. Histopathology of the telangiectasias associated with varicose veins. Dermatologia 127:321, 1963.

27. Wokalek H, Vanscheidt W, Martay K, Leder O. Morphology and localization of sunburst varicosities: an electron microscopic and morphometric study. J Dermatol Surg Oncol 15:149, 1989.

28. Barsky SH, Rosen S, Geer D, et al. The nature and evolution of port wine stains: a computer-assisted study. J Invest Dermatol 74:154, 1980.

29. Rosen S. Nature and evolution of port-wine stains. *In* Cutaneous Laser Therapy: Principles and Methods. Edited by Arndt KA, Noe JM, Rosen S. New York, John Wiley, 1983, pp 75–84.

30. Finley JL, Noe JM, Arndt KA, Rosen S. Port-wine stains. Morphologic variations and developmental lesions. Arch Dermatol 120:1453, 1984.

31. Apfelberg DB, Maser MR, Lash H, et al. Use of the argon and carbon dioxide lasers for treatment of superficial venous varicosities of the lower extremity. Lasers Surg Med 4:221, 1984.

32. Apfelberg DB, Smith T, Maser MR, et al. Study of three laser systems for treatment of superficial varicosities of the lower extremity. Lasers Surg Med 7:219, 1987.

33. Frazzetta M, Palumbo FP, Bellisi M, et al. Considerations regarding the use of the CO_2 laser: personal case study. Laser 2:4, 1989.

34. Landthaler M, Haina D, Waidelich W, Brown-Falco O. Laser therapy of venous lakes (Bean-Walsh) and telangiectasias. Plast Reconstr Surg 73:78, 1984.

35. Greenwald J, Rosen S, Anderson RR, et al. Comparative histological studies of the tunable dye (577nm) laser and argon laser: the specific vascular effects of the dye laser. J Invest Dermatol 77:305, 1981.

36. van Gemert MJC, Henning JPH. A model approach to laser coagulation of dermal vascular lesions. Arch Dermatol Res 270:429, 1981.

37. Finley JL, Arndt KA, Noe JM, Rosen S. Argon laser port-wine stain interaction: immediate effects. Arch Dermatol 120:613, 1984.

38. Arndt KA. Treatment technics in argon laser therapy: comparison of pulsed and continuous exposures. J Am Acad Dermatol 11:90, 1984.

39. Apfelberg DB, Maser MR, Lash H. Argon laser management of cutaneous vascular deformities—a preliminary report. West J Med 124:99, 1976.

40. Apfelberg DB, Flores JT, Maser MR, Lash H. Analysis of complications of argon laser treatment for port wine hemangiomas with reference to striped technique. Lasers Surg Med 2:357, 1983.

41. Apfelberg DB, Maser MR, Lash H. Treatment of nevi aranei by means of an argon laser. J Dermatol Surg Oncol 4:172, 1978.

42. Lyons GD, Owens RE, Mouney DF. Argon laser destruction of cutaneous telangiectatic lesions. Laryngoscope 91:1322, 1981.

43. Remington BK. Argon laser therapy—rosacea, telangiectasia (Letter to the editor). J Dermatol Surg Oncol 9:424, 1983.

44. Goldman L. Application of laser therapy. Paper given at the Noah Worcester Dermatologic Society, Hilton Head, April, 1984.

45. Arndt IA. Argon laser therapy of small cutaneous vascular lesions. Arch Dermatol 118:219, 1982.

46. Dixon JA, Huether S, Rotering RH. Hypertrophic scarring in argon laser treatment of port-wine stains. Plast Reconstr Surg 73:771, 1984.

47. Ratz JL, Goldman L, Bauman WE. Post treatment complications of the argon laser. Arch Dermatol 121:714, 1985.

48. Landthaler M, Haina D, Seipp W, et al. Argon laser treatment of naevi flammei. Hautarzt 38:652, 1987.

49. Olbricht SM, Stern RS, Tang SV, et al. Complications of cutaneous laser surgery: a survey. Arch Dermatol 123:345, 1987.

50. Bonafe JL, Laffitte F, Chavoin JP, et al. Hyperpigmentation induced by argon laser therapy of hemangiomas: optimal and electron microscope studies. Dermatologica 170:225, 1985.

51. Apfelberg DB, McBurney E. Use of the argon laser in dermatologic surgery. *In* Lasers in Cutaneous Medicine and Surgery. Edited by Ratz JL. Chicago, Year Book Medical Publishers Inc., 1986, pp 31–71.

52. Craig RDP, Purser JM, Lessells AM, Hufton AP. Argon laser therapy for cutaneous lesions. Br J Plast Surg 38:148, 1985.

53. Apfelberg DB, Maser MR, Lash H, et al. Use of the argon and carbon dioxide lasers for treatment of superficial venous varicosities of the lower extremity. Lasers Surg Med 4:221, 1984.

54. Dixon JA, Rotering RH, Huether SE. Patient's evaluation of argon laser therapy of port wine stain, decorative tattoo and essential telangiectasia. Lasers Surg Med 4:181, 1984.

55. Corcos L, Longo L. Classification and treatment of telangiectases of the lower limbs. Laser 1:22, 1988.

56. Tan OT, Murray S, Kurban AK. Action spectrum of vascular specific injury using pulsed irradiation. J Invest Dermatol 92:868, 1989.

57. Garden JM, Tan OT, Kerschmann R, et al. Effect of dye laser pulse duration on selective cutaneous vascular injury. J Invest Dermatol 87:653, 1986.

58. Tan OT, Carney JM, Margolis R, et al. Histologic responses of port-wine stains treated by argon, carbon dioxide, and tunable dye lasers: a preliminary report. Arch Dermatol 122:1016, 1986.

59. Tan OT, Sherwood K, Gilchrest BA. Treatment of children with port-wine stains using the flashlamp-pulsed tunable dye laser. N Engl J Med 320:416, 1989.

60. Garden JM, Tan OT, Parrish JA. The pulsed dye laser: its use at 577 nm wavelength. J Dermatol Surg Oncol 13:134, 1987.

61. Polla LL, Tan OT, Garden JM, Parrish JA. Tunable pulsed dye laser for the treatment of benign cutaneous vascular ectasia. Dermatologica 174:11, 1987.

62. Fajardo LF, Prionas SD, Kowalski J, Kwan HH. Hyperthermia inhibits angiogenesis. Radiat Res 114:297, 1988.

63. Goldman MP, Kaplan RP, Oki LN, et al. Sclerosing agents in the treatment of telangiectasia: comparison of the clinical and histologic effects of intravascular polidocanol, sodium tetradecyl sulfate, hypertonic saline in the dorsal rabbit ear vein model. Arch Dermatol 123:1196, 1987.

64. Biegeleisen K. Primary lower extremity telangiectasias—relationship of size to color. Angiology 38:760, 1987.

65. Ashton N. Corneal vascularization. *In* The Transparency of the Cornea. Edited by Duke-Elder S, Perkins ES. Oxford, Blackwell, 1960.

66. Folkman J, Klagsbrun M. Angiogenic factors. Science 235:442, 1987.

67. Ryan TJ. Factors influencing the growth of vascular endothelium in the skin. Br J Dermatol 82(suppl. 5):99, 1970.

68. Nakagawa H, Tan OT, Parrish JA. Ultrastructural changes in human skin after exposure to a pulsed laser. J Invest Dermatol 84:396, 1985.

69. Tan OT, Carney JM, Margolis R, et al. Histologic responses of port-wine stains treated by argon, carbon dioxide, and tunable dye lasers: a preliminary report. Arch Dermatol 122:1016, 1986.

70. Goldman MP, Martin DE, Fitzpatrick RE, Ruiz-Esparza J. Pulse dye laser treatment of telangiectasia with and without sub-therapeutic sclerotherapy: clinical and histologic examination in the rabbit ear vein model. J Am Acad Dermatol 23:23, 1990.

71. Dvorak HF. Tumors: Wounds that do not heal: similarities between tumor stroma generation and wound healing. N Engl J Med 315:1650, 1986.

72. Majewski S, Kaminski M, Jablonska S, et al. Angiogenic capability of peripheral blood mononuclear cells in psoriasis. Arch Dermatol 121:1018, 1985.

73. Goldman MP, Fitzpatrick RE. Pulsed-dye laser treatment of leg telangiectasia: with and without simultaneous sclerotherapy. J Dermatol Surg Oncol 16:338, 1990.

Chapter 14   Living With a Port-Wine Birthmark

Pina Clementina Masciarelli

The nonmedical causes of port-wine stain birthmarks: having an unmet craving for wine during pregnancy; eating bad strawberries during pregnancy; walking through a garden without shoes; dipping one's hand into red paint; eating hot peppers; getting too much/too little sun; being a "bad" child.

When I was first asked to write this chapter, my biggest concern was how long it needed to be. I kept putting it off. As I finally began writing it two weeks before the due date, I realized that my ambivalence had more to do with the overwhelming emotions connected with having this degenerative disorder.

I have a port-wine stain covering my upper right extremity including my arm, breast, and scapula area, never crossing the midline. The course of the disorder has reached the level where I have minimal-to-moderate loss in fine motor coordination, sensation, and strength in my upper extremity. Endurance is also limited. I have raised nodules throughout the involved area. The nail of my third digit has had repeated fungus and bacterial infections; I also have a swan-neck deformity in the peripheral joint of this finger. I wear a below-the-elbow Jobst glove to assist with the edema and to promote positive circulation. I should also add that I am right dominant and stubbornly so.

When I was born, the hemangioma covered a more extensive area and was a dark black-purple color. At first, the birthmark was not identified or understood—the prognosis was said to be unclear. My father saw me soon after birth, but it was not until two days later that I was brought to my mother. This delay occurred because no health care professional was able to identify the abnormality. Finally, a passing pediatrician recognized the birthmark for what it was.

Over the years, I have heard many "explanations" from professionals and nonprofessionals for my "red arm." Many of these bizarre reasonings have left me confused and speechless. Looking back now, I wonder where these interpretations came from. I realize, however, how they shaped my personal growth.

Pina Clementina Masciarelli is a Senior Occupational Therapist at the UMASS Adolescent Treatment Program at Westborough State Hospital, Westborough, MA. She also has a private practice specializing in mental health.

My right arm has always been larger in terms of its size rather than its length. My fingers are usually the size of Italian sausages. The earliest I remember them aching was when I was eight years old. My mother took me to a dermatologist who said not to worry because the entire birthmark would be gone by the time I was 16. When I was 14, I began to get sharp, hot pains in my hand. The involved area soon began to include my forearm, then my upper arm, and in recent years, my breast, shoulder, and scapula. There are also aches that nag for hours and interfere with my functional abilities.

Beyond the physical interferences in daily living, there is the emotional drain that affects my basic functioning. First, more than the pain, the swelling, and the numbness, there is the knowledge of loss of functioning— when I drop a cup of coffee because it's too heavy, when I cannot pick up a dime because my fingers cannot pinch such a fine object, not being able to take notes in class because I did paperwork during the day, not being able to carry an infant on my right side, and not knowing when I am being touched in an area even in a tender moment. It is a horrible experience when I realize that something I could do last week I can no longer do today.

Then, there is the emotional injury, the almost daily explanation to others, that is still unclear to me, of why I have a "red arm." From the time I was young, if I was not recognized by my name, the physical description often included was "she has a red arm." There was an endless list of names that I was called and ridiculed with. Children, because they have not had the experience of difference as their elders have had, often tease as a way of dealing with something that is not understood. Adults, however, who do have the capacity to understand, are often crueler in their remarks and comments. Defending my "color" got me into all sorts of mischief growing up—but I will leave those tales to my family, teachers, and peers.

In high school I was identified as "colored," with a negative connotation, but it gave me the opportunity to share in experiences with other races and accept myself more for who I was. In this regard my birthmark has had a positive influence on my character.

As an adult, I recognize more the discrimination that occurs with my disorder, whereas in childhood I thought that others' reactions were due to my being "defective." People refuse to shake my hand, they stand back away from me, they give odd looks out of the corner of their eyes, and they make inappropriate comments about something they do not understand. How does one explain the color of one's skin?

When I was in college, I commuted daily by train; there was an older woman who got on at Copley Station who I often gave my seat to. One day she got on the train with another woman. After I got up to give the woman my seat, I heard her say to the friend, "See, that was the girl I was telling you about, the one with the red hand." For the longest time after that I drove into school.

I have seen many doctors of different specialties and backgrounds, and I could go on and on describing just what physicians have told me was wrong with my arm. These explanations included that I had a "bad arm," "nothing to worry about," rheumatoid arthritis, Sturge-Weber syndrome, a spinal cord injury, or there was just nothing wrong. Although bits and pieces of these diagnoses were valid, they in no way explained the true process of what was occurring.

The worst week was the one before my twenty-fourth birthday. On Monday I was told by a respected physician that I needed to "face reality" and that my arm would soon become gangrenous and need to be amputated! On that Friday, I was told by a well-known laser surgeon that all that was happening in my arm was completely "psychological"! I was HORRIFIED!! Needless to say I did not have a good birthday that year. Shortly after that experience, I had a long discussion with my neurologist, who wisely explained that doctors' personalities not only influence the field of medicine they choose but also dictate how they react to what they do not know. I then took a break from trying to find out what was happening to me physically to work on my mental health.

The Laser Treatments

I should preface this section by stating that the experiences I describe regarding my birthmark and the laser treatments are my own, and the effects on others may be different. In discussing them here as in the rest of the chapter, they are meant to be informative to others and part of a healing process for myself.

I began laser treatments July 8, 1989. At this point, I have gone over most of the involved area at least once. I have tried to come up with creative nicknames for the laser treatments. My favorites are the "zapping" verb: "to zap, zapped, be zapped," etc.—and the "barbeque" verb: "to barbeque, barbequed, be barbequed," etc. The latter goes well with the summer motif.

It seems as though I am always going for laser treatments. There have been times when I have gone for treatments for seven weekends in a row. This is not because I am dedicated to the laser, but rather to my health. It is amazing how much energy the treatments take. For those considering giving and/or receiving the treatments, I have learned that there are certain things that could be done to make the therapy process easier.

First, it is important to plan ahead. For example, all errands should be done in advance—i.e., food shopping, purchasing of medical supplies, arranging for rides, doing laundry, ironing clothes, cooking dinners, opening jars.

There are two things that have helped me stay sane in going for these treatments. One of these is to do something good for myself before every treatment. It could be, and has been, anything imaginable—from getting my nails manicured to eating dessert before dinner to making a long-distance call to a good friend. It is amazing how these seemingly insignificant events have become so helpful in setting a positive frame of mind. I have also found that meeting individuals and families who also have port-wine stains and sharing experiences with them is a powerful tool in getting support.

The other incredibly helpful piece has been that I have taken a friend or family member to accompany me to every laser treatment. Their support and caring have made the procedure so much more bearable and the treatment more therapeutic. I cannot stress this enough, or thank enough those people who have been there for me, not only to make sure that I get to the appointments on time, but also to sit in the treatment sessions with me and make sure that I am comfortable and cared for after each procedure.

The treatments themselves hurt! Although I have heard them described as feeling like a rubber band snapping against the skin, to me it is more like someone is taking a hot rod and pressing it against my skin; and when it is repeated over and over in an area, I KNOW! What happens internally is another process. All the obscene phrases that I learned during adolescence come flooding back to mind—including the one that I never said! Depending on the sensitivity of the area treated, the intense pain has lasted from an hour after treatment to more than a day. Beyond that there is a feeling of soreness that eases with ice, an elevated position, and time. Initially changing the bandages and cleaning the area is also painful; but this also decreases as the area heals.

What has helped me during the treatment procedure is to be focused on something else. I am always aware of the laser, but it helps to be involved in another activity. My distraction has always been to talk and keep talking. We have had some whimsical and intense discussions during my treatments—pity the man who walks into the treatment room during one of the all-female sessions. There are times during the treatments when I have become light-headed and have felt disorganized; I think this may be my body's personal reaction to the laser. When I do feel this way, it is helpful even if I am not participating in the discussion to have those around me talking to distract me from the treatment procedure. Again, I cannot thank enough all those people who have been there for me to get me through the treatments.

My disorganization sometimes lasts for a short time after the treatments, so that I do not always have a high morale. Just as it is important to do something good for myself before the treatments, it is necessary to do something esteem-building afterwards. For me, ice cream has always worked—it is amazing what a double chocolate waffle cone with mud pie ice cream can do for my level of comfort! Or a walk in the park or even a ride to the beach—and all of these include a carry-on ice pack, of course.

It does take a few days to recover and to return to somewhat routine functioning. Even when the treated area heals on the exterior level, there seems to be a longer recovery process occurring internally that makes resuming normal activities a lengthier process. The bandages and packing do not make for the most attractive outerwear, especially when the padding necessary for edema and protection is in places that are not usually lumpy. Also when my hand or forearm has been treated it has been helpful for edema to wear a splint for support, and to use elevation during the day and at times at night. This period of immobilization has tried my patience on many occasions and has not made me one of the most tranquil people to be around. However, it has made my healing process much more therapeutic.

During the post-treatment process, there are a few protocols to follow, including: no aspirin (no problem, many nonaspirin products exist); no alcohol (I easily skip that); and no aerobics (ouch!). Because of increased blood flow caused by exercise, the treated area can be damaged by intense workouts; I have had to find new ways of working out and letting go of my tension. My vice continues to be the sun. Although I use Photoplex faithfully on the involved area, I am a sun lover—this has not scored me points with my physician.

Because my birthmark is so extensive, there are times when cleaning and putting on fresh bandages are quite awkward. I have gotten myself into the strangest positions just to put on Bacitracin—it is not a pretty sight. Then there are the Telfa bandages, gauze, tape, Kling, Ace; some days more of these end up in the wastebasket than on me. I come out looking pretty strange, too. A little bit of Ace here, a splint there, some gauze sticking out from under this or that, plus all the bulges from areas that are usually hidden from the public eye. The first time I received a treatment on my breast, I looked down and saw this huge, knobby 38DDD breast on the right and a little 34C on the left. That's when I started to wear the big bulky sweaters after treatments.

A Clinician's Perspective

Being an occupational therapist has been helpful in adapting my environment and lifestyle to the disease and treatments. On the other hand, I know too much—like the rheumatologist being treated for rheumatoid arthritis, or a dentist having chronic gum disease. The emotional impact of being a health professional is another area that I have needed to recognize and address in my healing process.

As an occupational therapist, I find myself on both sides of the fence. I am a patient with a disease that interferes with my daily living. On the other hand, I am a clinician trained to assess not only the physical abilities of a person, but also the emotional and occupational status—i.e., the whole person. In some respects this dual role has helped me understand my disorder and treatments more clearly; however, my daily analysis at times has raised my anxiety to new levels. It is devastating to recognize a loss in fine motor coordination or endurance and not have the immediate cure-all.

I am fortunate to have my own occupational therapist whom I see for treatment. I have daily prescribed exercises for strengthening and coordination. I am evaluated on a three-month basis in these areas to monitor the progress and adjust the treatment as needed. My therapist has also been helpful in suggesting ways to adapt myself and the environment to more functional daily living, including recommending strengthening exercises, the Jobst glove, and energy-conservation techniques.

Words of Wisdom

While writing this chapter, I have addressed personal issues that have been dormant or ignored for years. Looking at them now has helped me refocus my priorities and needs.

I have some comments I would like to share with the individuals, families, and treaters involved with port-wine stain birthmarks. First to my peers no matter what the age, I encourage you to seek treatment so that you may care for your total self. Address your physical needs as well as your emotional ones so that you may care for your whole person—you deserve it. And remember what Martin Luther King envisioned, that people should not be judged by the color of their skin but instead by what is inside the person.

I cannot stress enough to adults that they need to work out for themselves their issues around difference and individualism. For it is adults who set the pace not only for how others perceive someone with a port-wine stain (or any other disorder/difference), but also for how individuals, especially children, with the port-wine stains appreciate themselves.

For the families, especially the parents, I hope you can recognize that this birthmark is not caused by something you did, did not do, wished or wanted.

Recent research has not been able to detect the underlying cause of this disorder. What is known, however, is that it is a biological factor. I encourage you to talk to other families who share similar experiences so that you can be supported.

To the health care professionals, especially the physicians, I hope you will continue your research and treatment in this area. Further, I encourage you to look at yourselves and how you address what you do and do not know, and more importantly how this affects what you tell a patient. You may be creating an emotional scar that will have lasting effects. Also, utilize other disciplines so that you can treat the whole individual.

Today I was in the market. There were two women beside me; one said to the other, "Look, that woman has a fake hand"!

Index

Page numbers in italics indicate figures; numbers followed by "t" indicate tables.